I Can't Be Bothered COOKING

Edition 1

A Recipe Collection For When You Need Food
But Can't Be Bothered Cooking.

M. J. Adams

I Can't Be Bothered Cooking
Edition 1

Copyright M. J. Adams © 2025

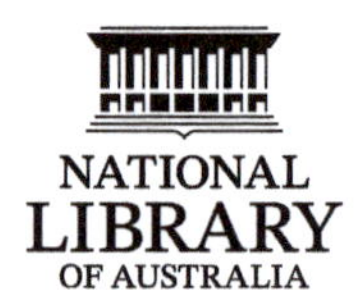

A catalogue record for this book is available from the National Library of Australia

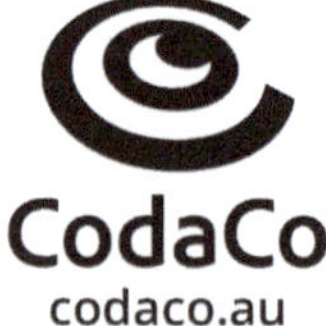

CodaCo
codaco.au

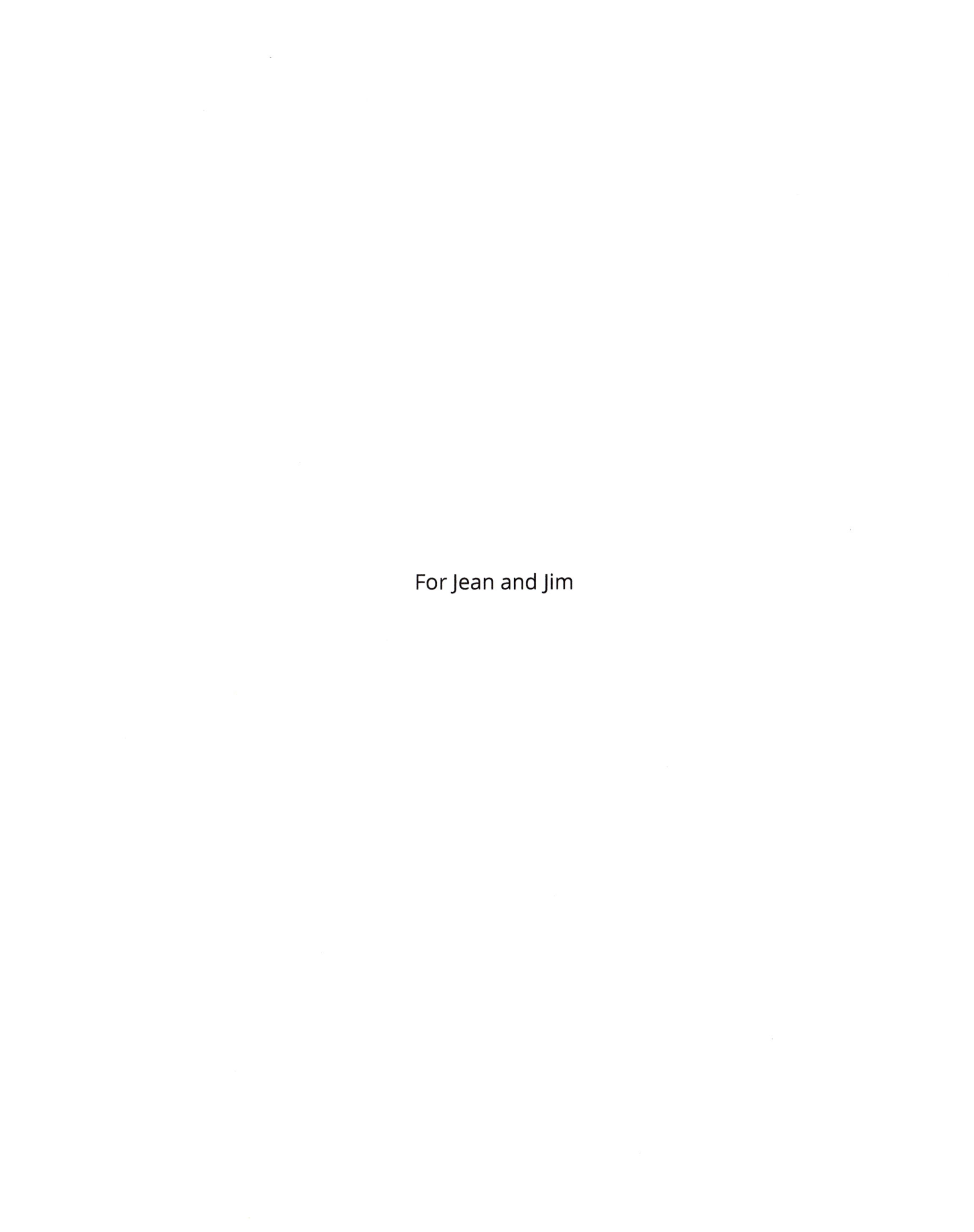

For Jean and Jim

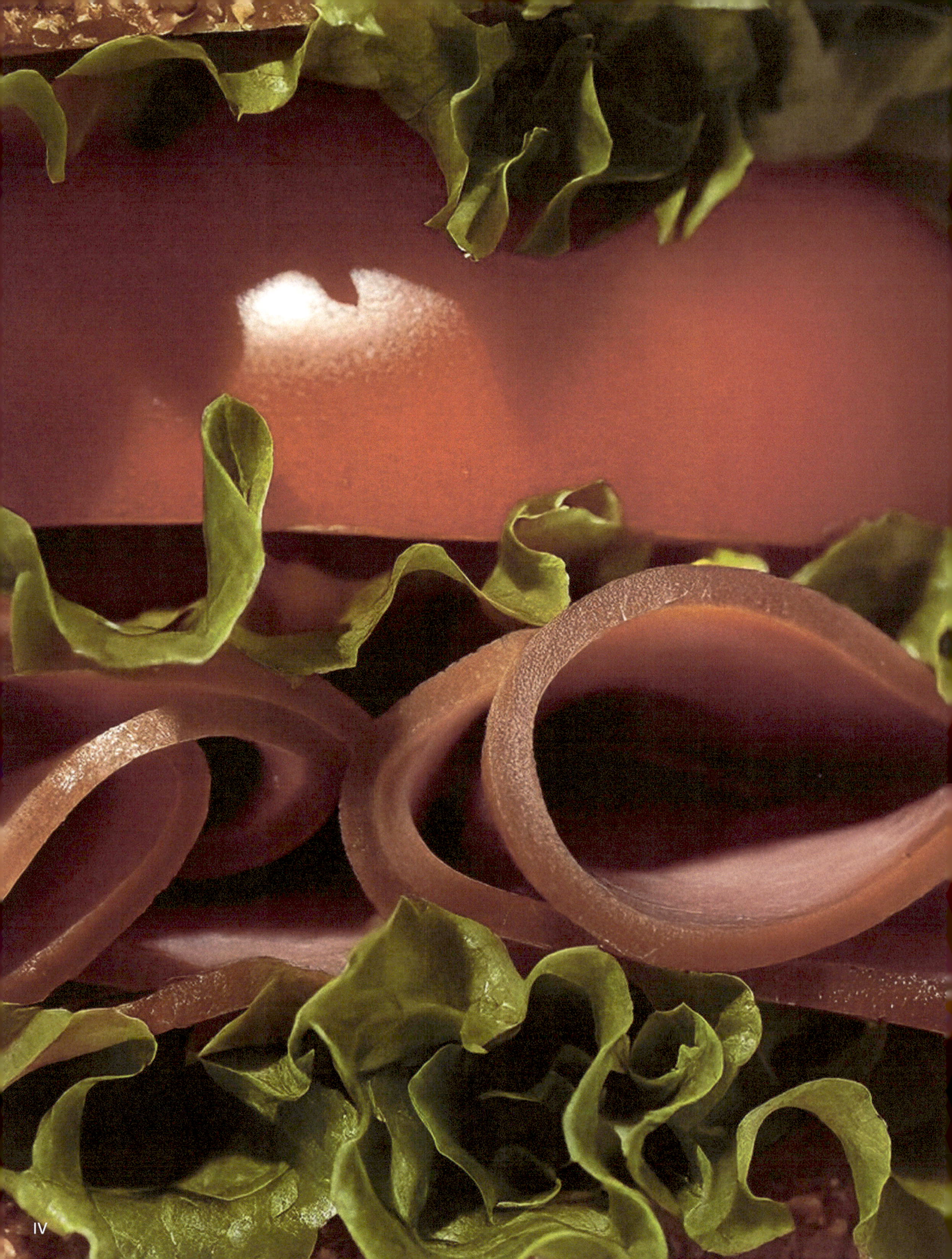

Table Of Contents

Preface

This book exists because many of us live in the real world, it's busy and relentless.

You know those moments

You're staring into your fridge at 8:47 PM after a 12 hour workday, your brain running on fumes, and the idea of chopping vegetables feels like climbing Mount Everest. Or it's Tuesday morning, you overslept, and you need breakfast that doesn't involve standing over a stove. Maybe you just got home from a night out, your head is pounding, and you need food that won't require actual thought because thinking hurts.

This isn't another cookbook promising you'll become a culinary genius. This is a survival guide for busy humans who need to eat good food but can't always muster the energy to prep, cook and cleanup. These are recipe food solutions for busy single people struggling with day to day nutrition.

Why This Book Can Help You

When you're running your own business while restoring a house and living without a kitchen or a working parent juggling soccer practice and client calls, you don't need a recipe that takes 45 minutes and dirties every pot in your kitchen. You need a breakfast that you can assemble in 15 minutes while your coffee brews because you have to be at work shortly.

When you're a college student surviving on loans and caffeine, you don't need ingredients that cost more than your textbooks. You need to know that the "The Leftover Club Sandwich" can be made from literally anything in your fridge and being agile with recipes is a survival technique.

When you're pulling an all nighter at work and it's 2 AM, you don't need a meal that requires planning, preparation or cleanup.

Real Situations, Real Solutions

Sunday Night Prep for the week: Spend 20 minutes cooking some rice and put it in the fridge. Now you can throw together salads, rice bowls, or wraps for the next few days without thinking. Using simple recipes, make your own pickles, spice blends and marinades for BBQ food so you can always have variety.

Simple, Fresh, Good

Every recipe in this book follows the same philosophy: maximum satisfaction with minimum effort made with fresh and frozen ingredients you already have. Nothing requires special equipment beyond a microwave and maybe a pan. Cleanup is minimal because nobody has time for that.

The Beauty of Minimal Prep

These aren't just recipes, they're recipe templates. Once you master the "basic wrap formula" or "rice bowl assembly," you can improvise based on whatever is available. It's cooking with minimal prep and cleanup.

Your Kitchen Rules

This book assumes you're a real person with a real life. Maybe you forgot to grocery shop. Maybe you only have three clean plates. Maybe you're eating dinner at 10 PM while binge watching Netflix or more likely you've been working all night. No judgment here.

Food doesn't have to be Instagram worthy to be satisfying. Sometimes a really good sandwich at midnight hits differently than a restaurant meal. Sometimes cereal for dinner is exactly what your body and soul needs. I've been there so many times.

Bottom Line

Life is complicated enough without stressing about every meal. You work hard, you're busy, and you deserve to eat something decent without turning it into a major production. The recipes take shortcuts because we are all busy, using pre-made ingredients, and prioritise convenience over perfection.

Because at the end of the day, fed is better than hungry. And sometimes the best meal is the one that requires the least effort. Simple is good and the fresher the food source is the better. We have to stop feeling guilty about all our food choices and when you should eat what. With these recipes you can make something delicious without all the prep and cleanup so you can get on with your life.

Introduction

We've all been there, it's 7 PM, you've been working all day, you're hungry, and the thought of actually cooking makes you want to order takeout for the fifth time this week. This book is for those moments when you need real food but your motivation is somewhere between zero and maybe tomorrow. This is especially relevant when dishes, pans and bowls fill the sink.

No complex techniques. No ingredient lists that read like a chemistry textbook. Just simple, satisfying meals that require minimal brain power, minimal prep and even less cleanup. Each recipe serves 1 and can be easily scaled up for more.

There is a shopping list at the end with key ingredients considered to be the basics for establishing a pantry.

No Time For Any Of This?

This Book Is For You And Someone You Know.

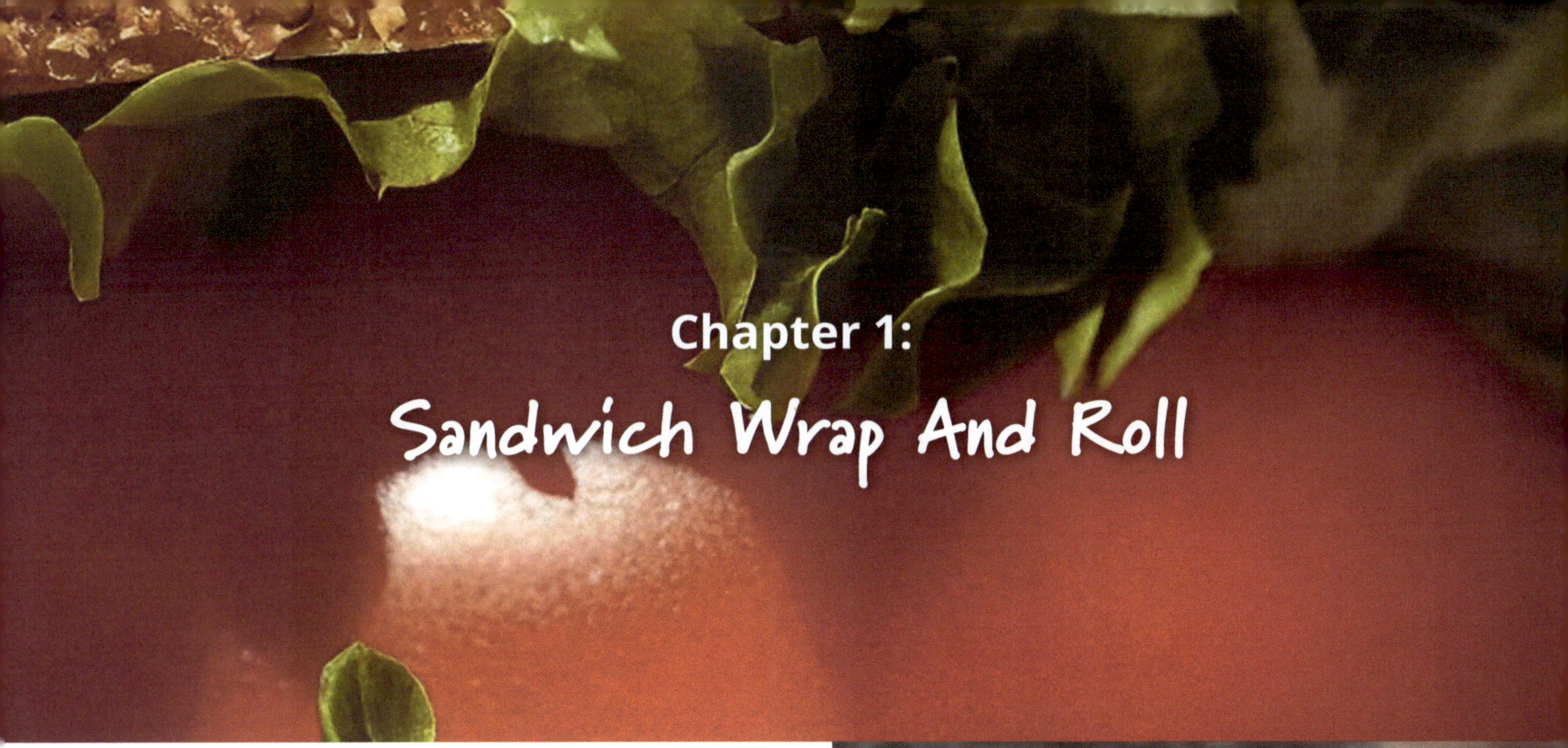

Chapter 1

Sandwich Wrap And Roll

The Leftover Club Sandwich

Time: 10 minutes

- 2 slices bread (wholemeal)
- Leftover meat chicken, ham, turkey
- Cheese slices
- Lettuce
- Sliced tomato
- Mayo or hot English mustard
- Onion sliced or pickle

Spread mayo or mustard over bread slices, stack it all together and move on.

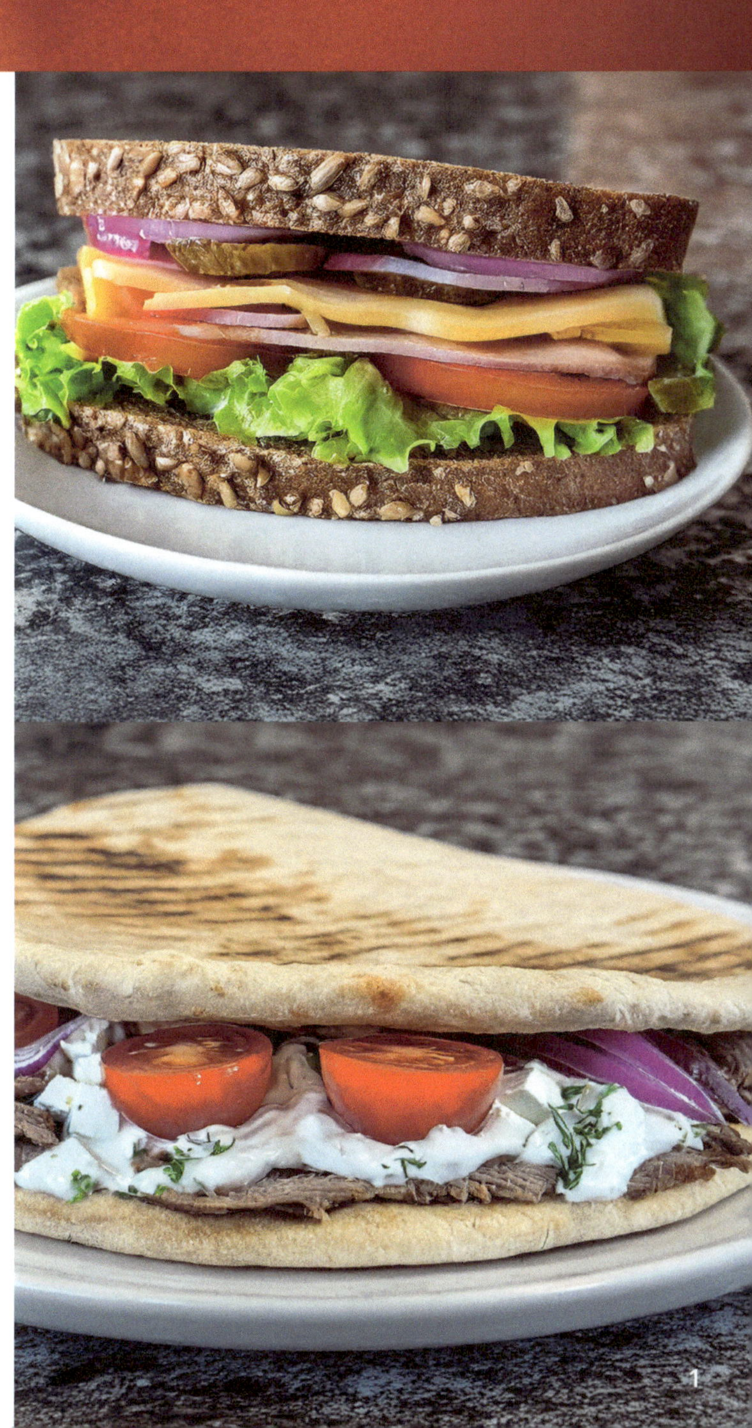

Mediterranean Lamb Pita

Time: 15 minutes

- 2 pita bread halves (1 large pita, warmed)
- 4 oz leftover roast lamb or chicken sliced thin
- 3 tbsp tzatziki sauce (store-bought is fine)
- 1/4 cucumber, diced
- 2 tbsp red onion, diced
- 3 cherry tomatoes, halved
- 3 tbsp crumbled feta cheese

Warm pita bread. Spread tzatziki inside pita and add lamb. Add onion, tomatoes and feta, drizzle olive oil and fold over.

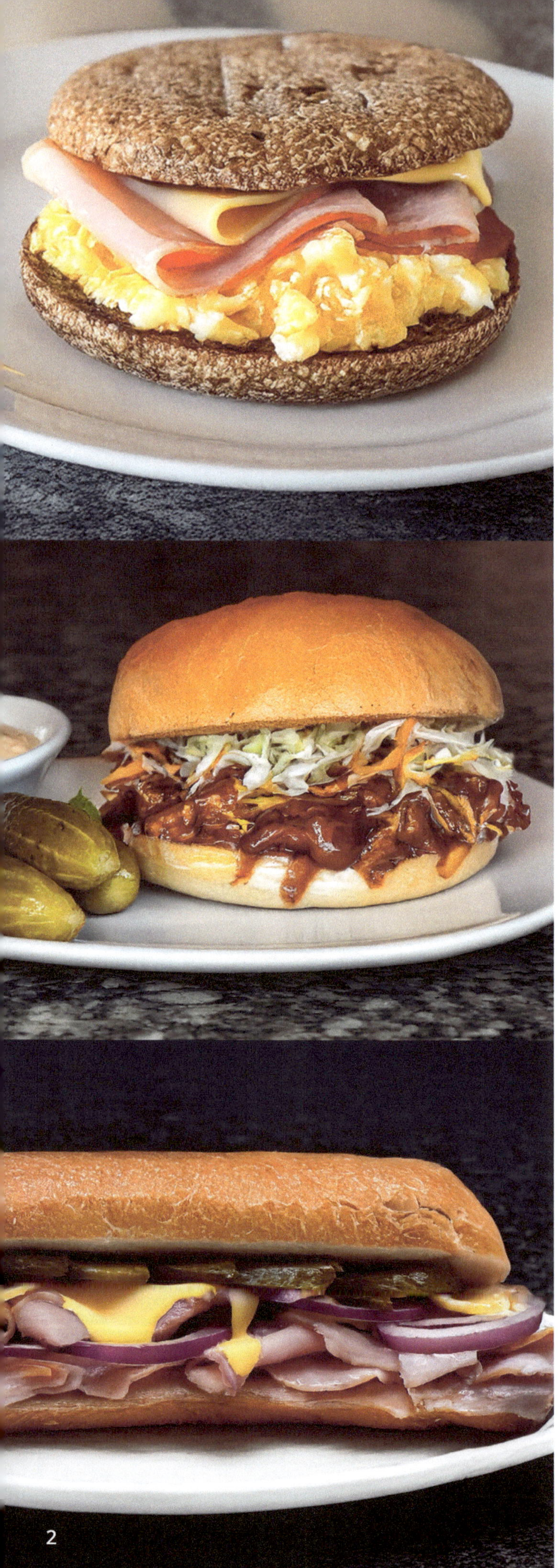

The Breakfast Sandwich

Time: 10 minutes

- English muffin or bagel
- 1 egg
- Cheese slice
- Bacon or ham slices
- Butter
- Black pepper or Everything seasoning (p15)

Cook egg however (scrambled is fastest). Toast muffin. Stack everything with cheese on top with cracked pepper and eat while hot.

BBQ Pulled Pork Roll

Time: 10 minutes (if you have leftover pork)

- Bread roll
- Leftover pulled pork or rotisserie chicken
- BBQ sauce
- Coleslaw mix (pre-made)
- Optional: Pickles

Heat meat with microwave and add BBQ sauce. Put on roll. Top with coleslaw. Add pickles for a tart contrast.

The Mojo Ham Sub

Time: 10 minutes

- 1 crusty sub roll
- 7 oz sliced ham (honey ham) or roast pork
- Sliced pickles and red onion
- 3 slices Swiss cheese with pickles
- Yellow hot mustard
- 1 tbsp butter, softened
- 1 tbsp mayonnaise

Slice sub lengthwise. Spread mustard on bottom and mayo on top. Add pork or ham, pickles and onion. Cook sub in pan with butter on both sides.

Tuna Melt for Lazy Days

Time: 8 minutes

- 1 can tuna
- 2 slices bread (any kind)
- Cheese slice
- Mayo (keep it minimal)
- Pickle
- Lemon Pepper seasoning

Mix tuna with mayo. Put on bread with cheese. Toast in toaster oven or in a pan until cheese melts. Done.

Grilled Cheese Plus

Time: 12 minutes

- 2 slices bread
- 4 cheese slices
- Ham
- Spinach
- Butter
- Optional: turkey, sliced apple

Butter outside of bread. Put cheese, spinach and ham inside. Cook in pan until golden and melted. Cut diagonally because you're not an animal.

BLT Without the Drama

Time: 15 minutes

- 2 slices bread (toasted)
- 4 strips bacon (pre-cooked or microwave)
- Lettuce
- Tomato slices
- Mayo
- Optional: avocado (recommended)

Toast bread. Cook bacon in a pan (or use pre-cooked). Stack it all up with bacon on top and enjoy. Simple perfection.

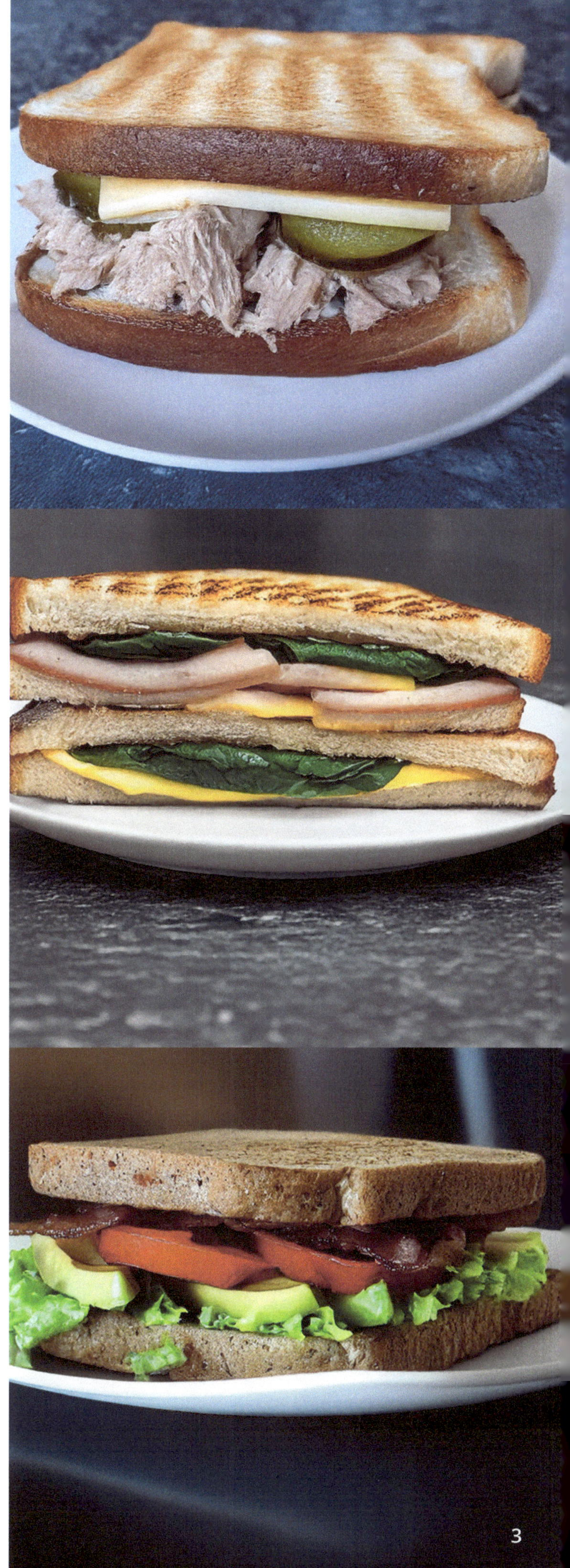

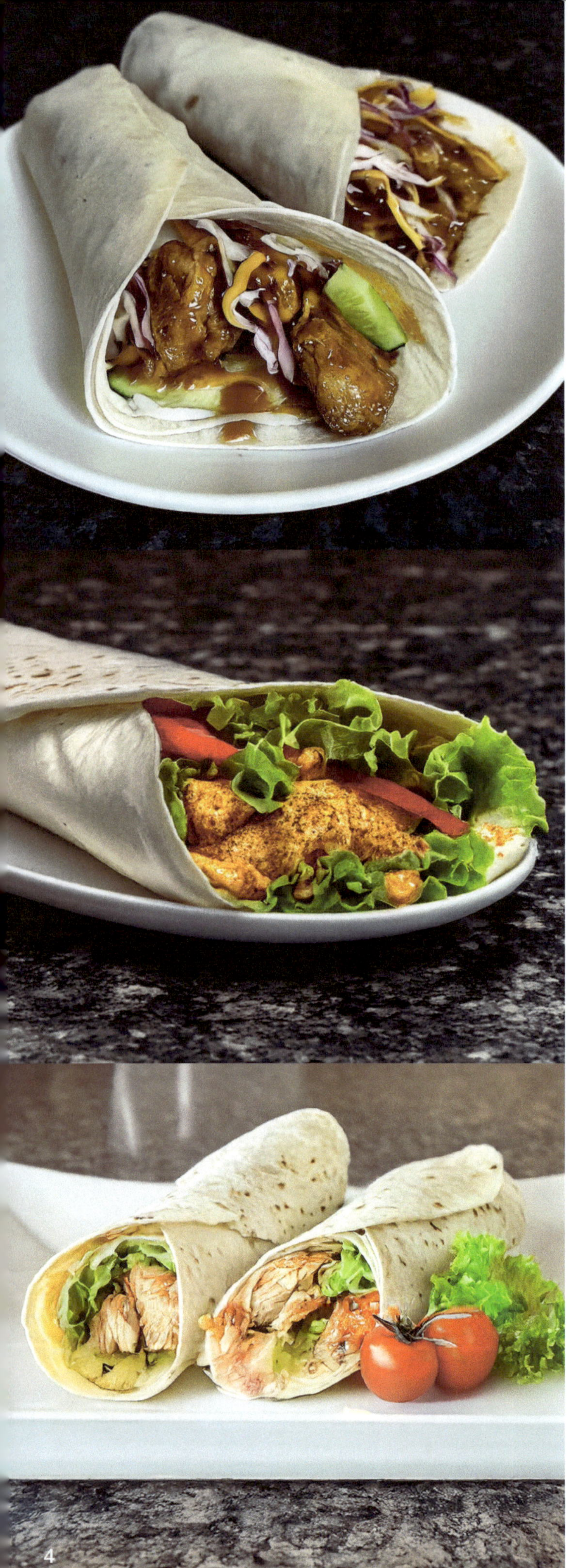

The Chicken Satay Wrap

Time: 8 minutes

- Plain tortilla (spinach or regular)
- 1 cup rotisserie chicken, shredded
- 3 tbsp peanut butter
- 1 tbsp soy sauce
- 1 tsp honey
- 1/2 tsp garlic powder
- 1/2 cup shredded coleslaw mix

Mix chicken pieces with everything in a bowl. Lay tortilla flat and spread mixture. Roll up and eat.

The Leftover Wrap

Time: 12 minutes

- Plain tortilla or flat bread
- Hummus or cream cheese spread
- Any combination: deli meat, leftover chicken
- Cheese
- Lettuce
- Tomato
- Peppers
- Hot sauce or Tabasco

Spread the base. Add all the good stuff. Roll tight.

Chicken Wrap

Time: 8 minutes

- Plain tortilla or flat bread
- Rotisserie chicken (shredded)
- Tabasco sauce
- Caesar dressing
- Lettuce
- Tomato

Mix chicken with Tabasco sauce. Spread Caesar dressing on tortilla/bread. Add chicken, tomato and lettuce. Roll up. Pretend you're at a sports bar.

Chicken Ranch Wrap

Time: 8 minutes

- Plain tortilla or flat bread
- Rotisserie chicken, shredded
- Caesar dressing
- Lettuce
- Shredded cheese
- Bacon bits

Mix chicken with ranch. Spread on tortilla with lettuce and cheese. Add bacon bits if available. Roll tight. Cut in half. Classic for a reason.

Mediterranean Veggie Wrap

Time: 6 minutes

- Plain tortilla or flat bread
- Hummus
- Cucumber and tomato slices
- Red onion
- Feta cheese
- Olives if you have them
- Spinach or lettuce

Spread hummus. Layer veggies mixed with feta cheese. Roll up, eat and enjoy.

Turkey Avocado Wrap

Time: 8 minutes

- Spinach and herb tortilla
- Spinach or lettuce
- Sliced turkey
- 1/2 avocado, sliced or mashed
- Cucumber slices
- Salt and pepper
- Optional: bacon bits, cheese

Slice or mash avocado with salt and pepper. Add spinach or lettuce, turkey and cucumber. Roll up. Actually tastes healthy.

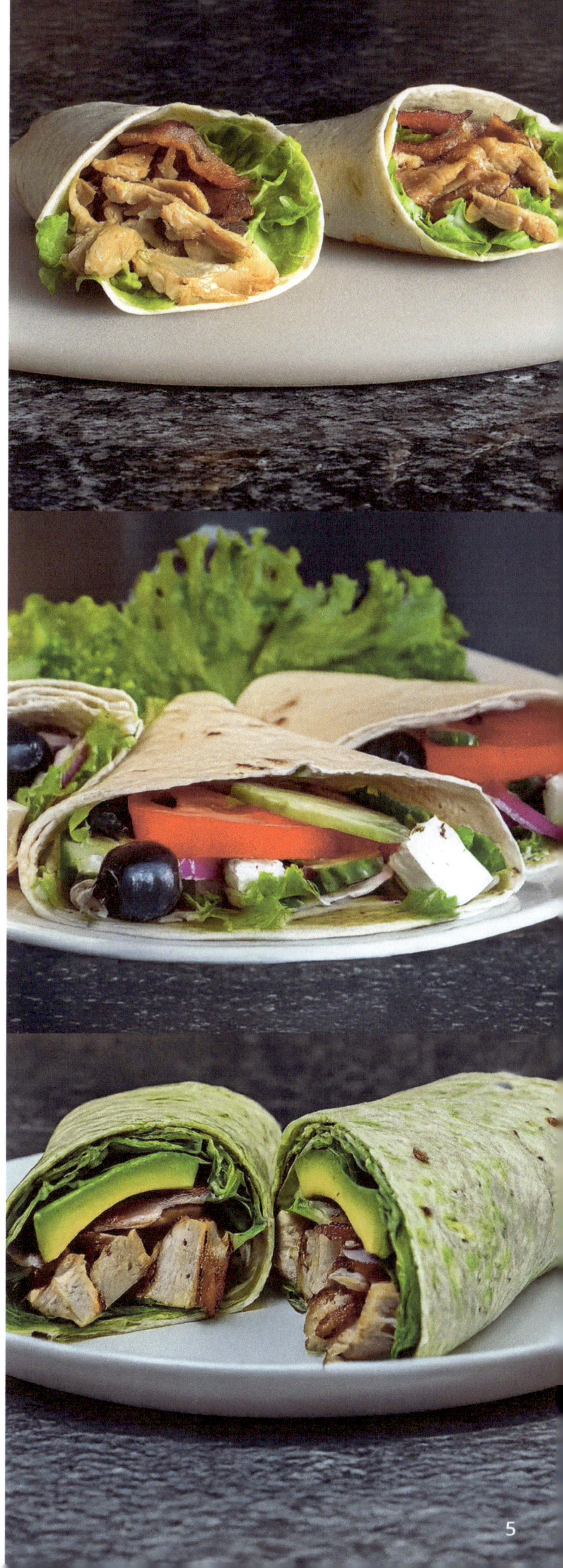

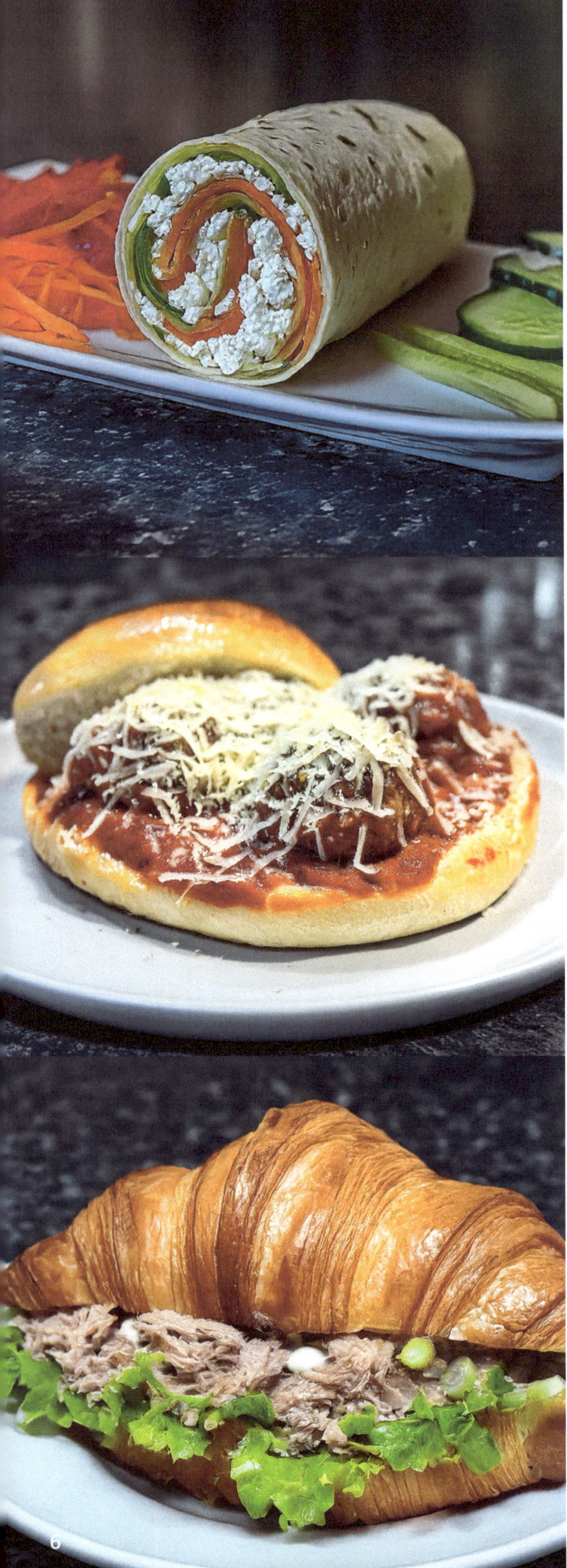

Veggie Cream Cheese Wrap

Time: 8 minutes

- Tortilla (spinach / regular)
- Cream cheese, softened
- Cucumber, julienned
- Black pepper
- Shredded carrots
- Cottage cheese

Spread cream cheese add cottage cheese. Add veggies in strips. Sprinkle black pepper. Roll tight. Slice in half if you want to eat it slower.

Meatball Marinara Roll

Time: 10 minutes

- Bread roll or sub
- Frozen meatballs
- Marinara sauce
- Mozzarella cheese
- Parmesan cheese
- Italian Blend seasoning

Microwave meatballs with sauce. Stuff in roll. Top with cheese. Toast until meatballs are hot and cheese is melted. Sprinkle seasoning and Parmesan.

Tuna Salad Croissant

Time: 10 minutes

- Croissant
- Canned tuna
- Mayo
- Diced celery (optional)
- Salt and pepper
- Lettuce

Mix tuna with mayo and seasonings. Add celery if you have it. Stuff in a cut croissant with lettuce. Cosmopolitan food without trying.

Roast Beef and Horseradish Roll

Time: 10 minutes

- Bread roll or thick crusty sub
- Sliced roast beef
- Horseradish sauce
- Lettuce
- Swiss cheese
- Tomato

Spread horseradish on roll. Layer beef, cheese, and greens. Add tomato and a spread of mustard if desired. Simple with a kick.

Italian Sub Roll

Time: 10 minutes

- Sub bread roll
- Salami, pepperoni, ham
- Provolone cheese or tasty matured
- Lettuce, tomato, onion
- Italian dressing (Edition 2)
- Optional: pickles, peppers

Layer meats and cheese. Add veggies. Drizzle dressing. Press down slightly. Eat over the sink like a civilized person.

Chicken Caesar Roll

Time: 10 minutes

- Crusty bread roll
- Rotisserie chicken
- Caesar dressing
- Lettuce
- Parmesan cheese
- Optional: croutons for crunch

Mix chicken with Caesar dressing. Stuff in roll with lettuce. Sprinkle cheese. Eat immediately.

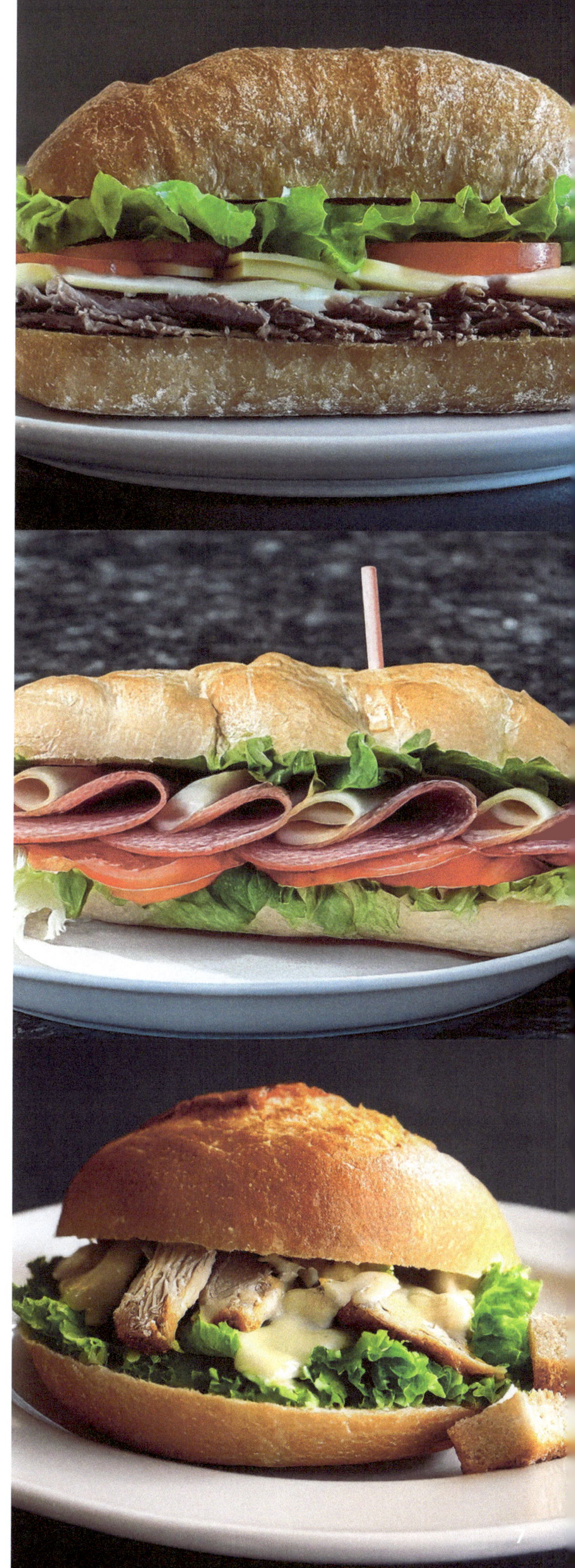

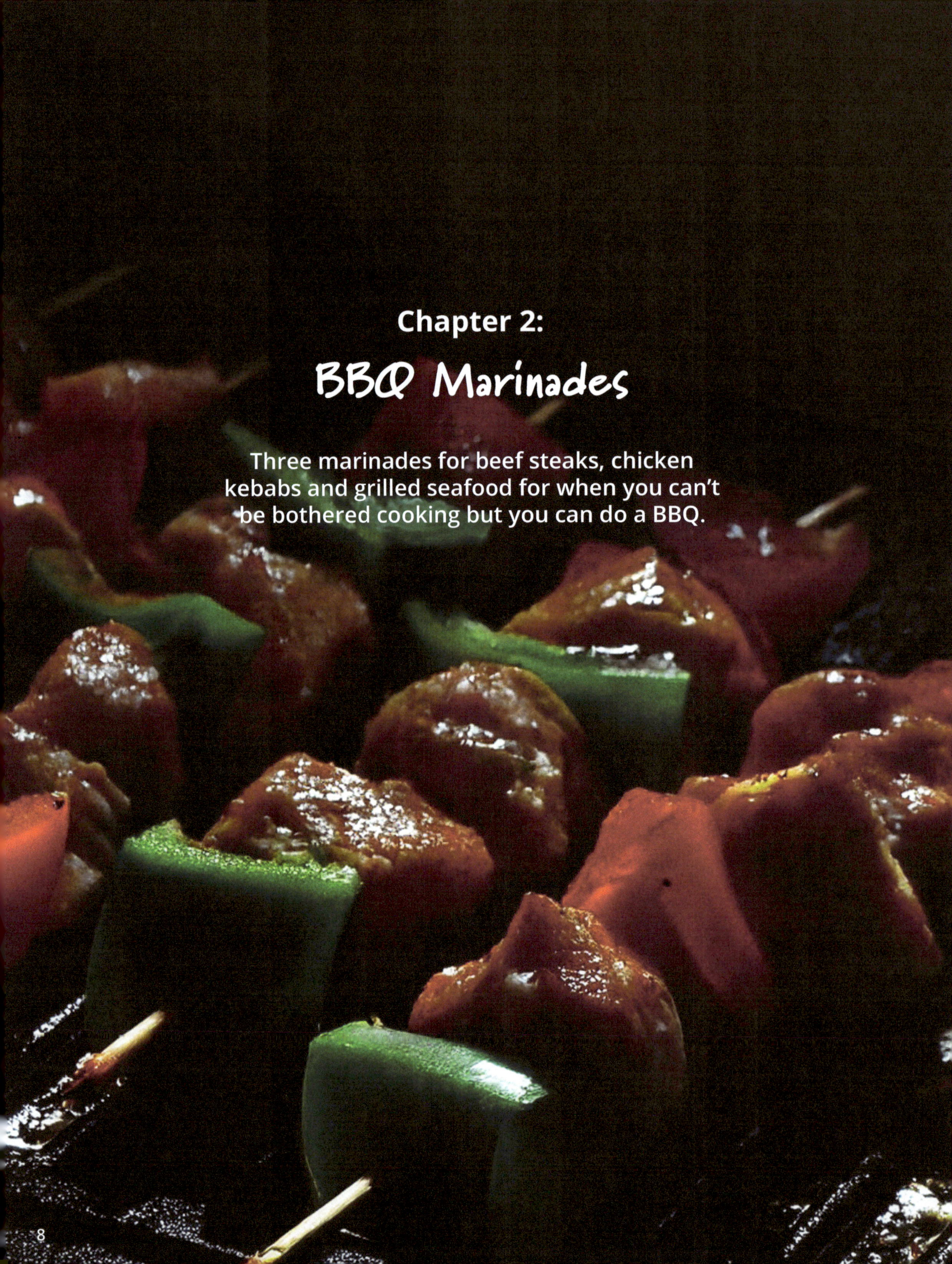

Chapter 2:
BBQ Marinades

Three marinades for beef steaks, chicken
kebabs and grilled seafood for when you can't
be bothered cooking but you can do a BBQ.

BBQ Steak Marinade

Perfect for beef steaks, this bold marinade
tenderizes and infuses deep, savory flavours.

- 1/4 cup soy sauce
- 1/4 cup olive oil
- 3 tablespoons Worcestershire sauce
- 2 tablespoons balsamic vinegar
- 4 cloves garlic, minced
- 1 teaspoon black pepper

Mix all ingredients and marinade beef steaks for
6-8hrs before BBQ. Brush marinade on while
cooking.

BBQ Lemon Marinade

A bright, Mediterranean inspired marinade keeps
chicken moist and delicious on the BBQ grill.

- 1/3 cup olive oil
- 1/4 cup fresh lemon juice (about 2 lemons)
- 3 cloves garlic, minced
- 2 tablespoons fresh oregano
- 1 tablespoon honey
- 1 teaspoon salt

Mix all ingredients and marinade cut chicken
pieces for 2hrs before BBQ. Brush marinade on
kebabs while cooking.

BBQ Seafood Marinade

A light, zesty marinade perfect for all seafood or
mixed seafood skewers.

- 3 tablespoons sesame oil
- 3 tablespoons soy sauce
- 2 tablespoons fresh lime or lemon juice
- 1 tablespoon honey
- 1 tablespoon sesame seeds
- 2 cloves garlic, minced

Mix all ingredients and marinade seafood for
30mins. Brush on marinade while cooking.

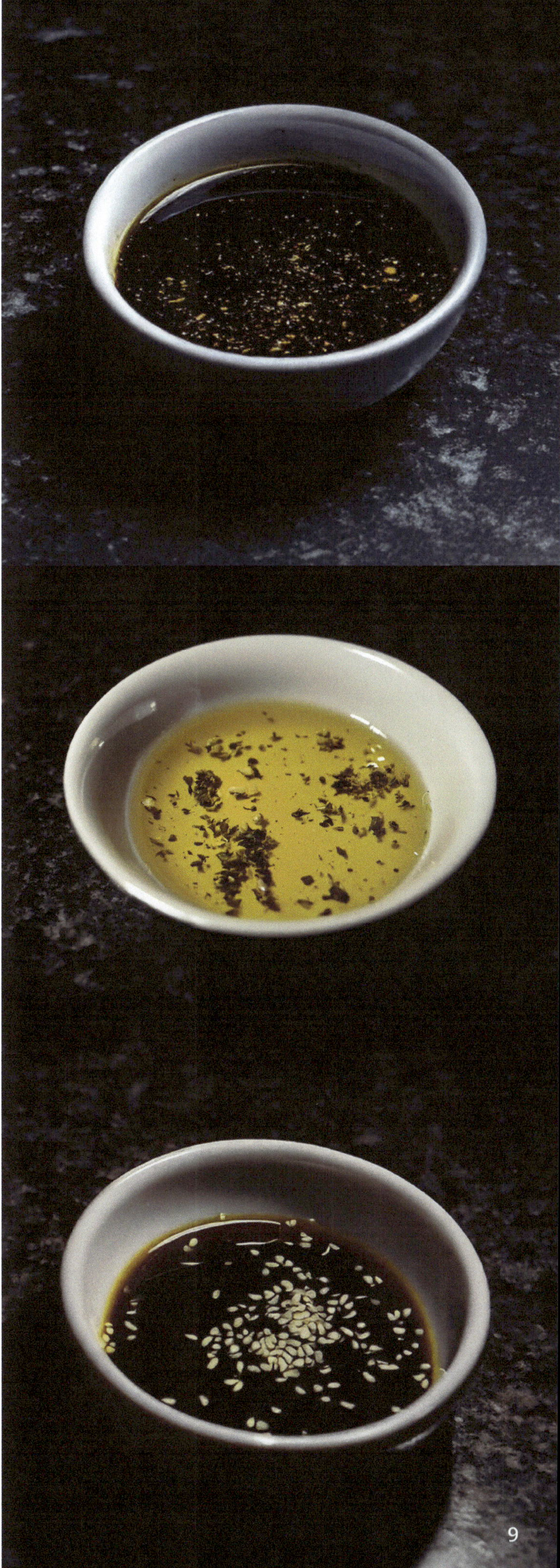

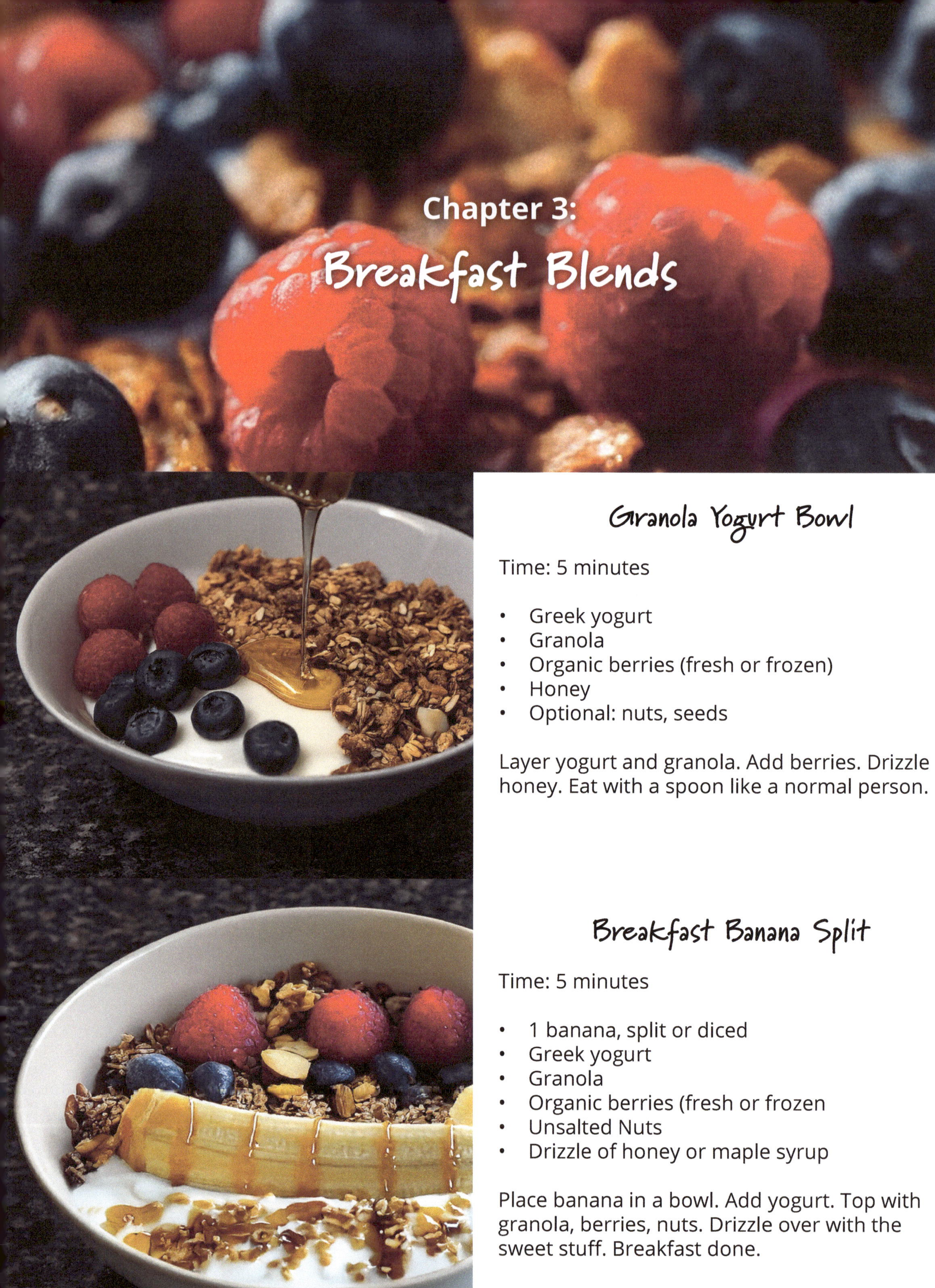

Chapter 3

Breakfast Blends

Granola Yogurt Bowl

Time: 5 minutes

- Greek yogurt
- Granola
- Organic berries (fresh or frozen)
- Honey
- Optional: nuts, seeds

Layer yogurt and granola. Add berries. Drizzle honey. Eat with a spoon like a normal person.

Breakfast Banana Split

Time: 5 minutes

- 1 banana, split or diced
- Greek yogurt
- Granola
- Organic berries (fresh or frozen
- Unsalted Nuts
- Drizzle of honey or maple syrup

Place banana in a bowl. Add yogurt. Top with granola, berries, nuts. Drizzle over with the sweet stuff. Breakfast done.

Overnight Oats (Prepare Day Before)

Time: 6 minutes prep, overnight wait

- 1/2 cup oats
- 1/2 cup milk
- 1 tbsp Chia seeds
- Maple syrup or honey
- Vanilla extract
- Toppings: nuts, berries and fruit

Mix everything except toppings in jar. Refrigerate overnight. Add toppings in morning. Eat cold.

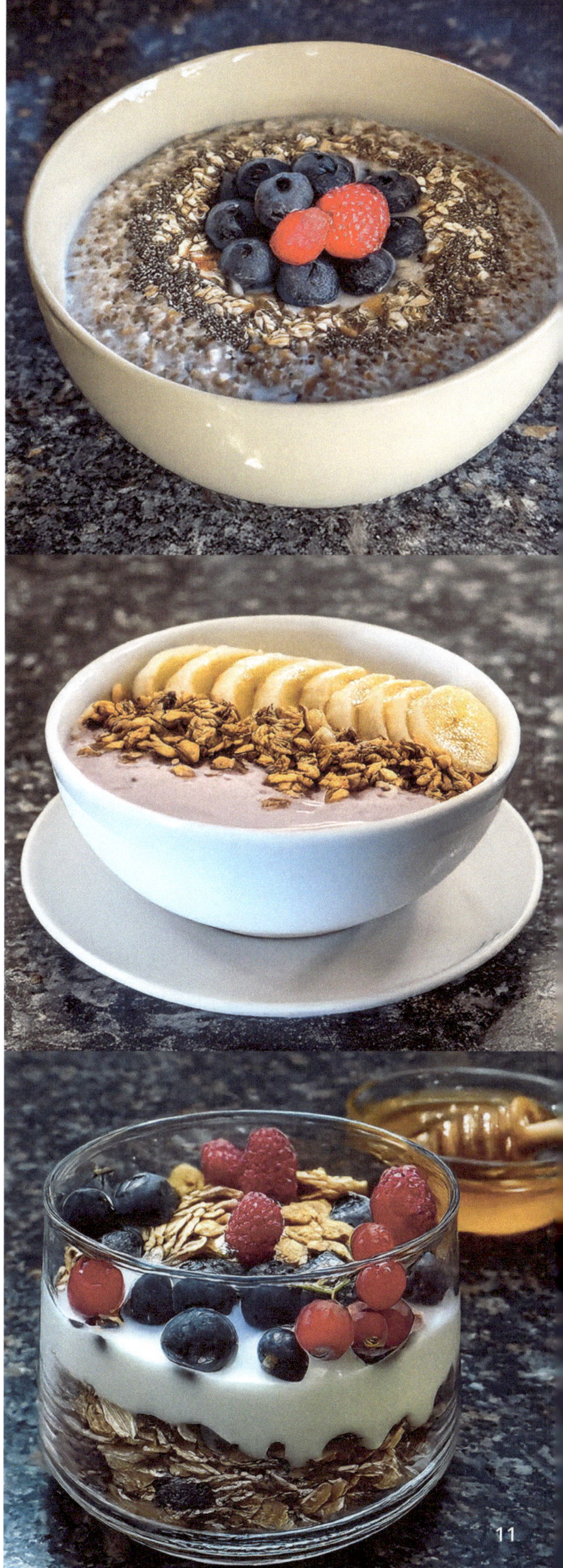

Cheyenne Smoothie

Time: 5 minutes

- Organic berries (fresh or frozen)
- Banana
- Splash of dairy milk or tiger nut milk or juice
- Granola for topping
- Optional: protein powder (you won't taste it)

Blend frozen stuff with milk or juice until thick. Pour in a bowl. Add granola. Eat slowly with a spoon while feeling healthy and virtuous then move on with your day.

Cereal Parfait

Time: 5 minutes

- Your favorite cereal
- Greek yogurt
- Organic berries (fresh or frozen)
- Honey
- Optional: Unsalted cashews

Layer yogurt, cereal, and berries in a glass or bowl. Drizzle honey. Repeat layers. Eat immediately before cereal gets soggy.

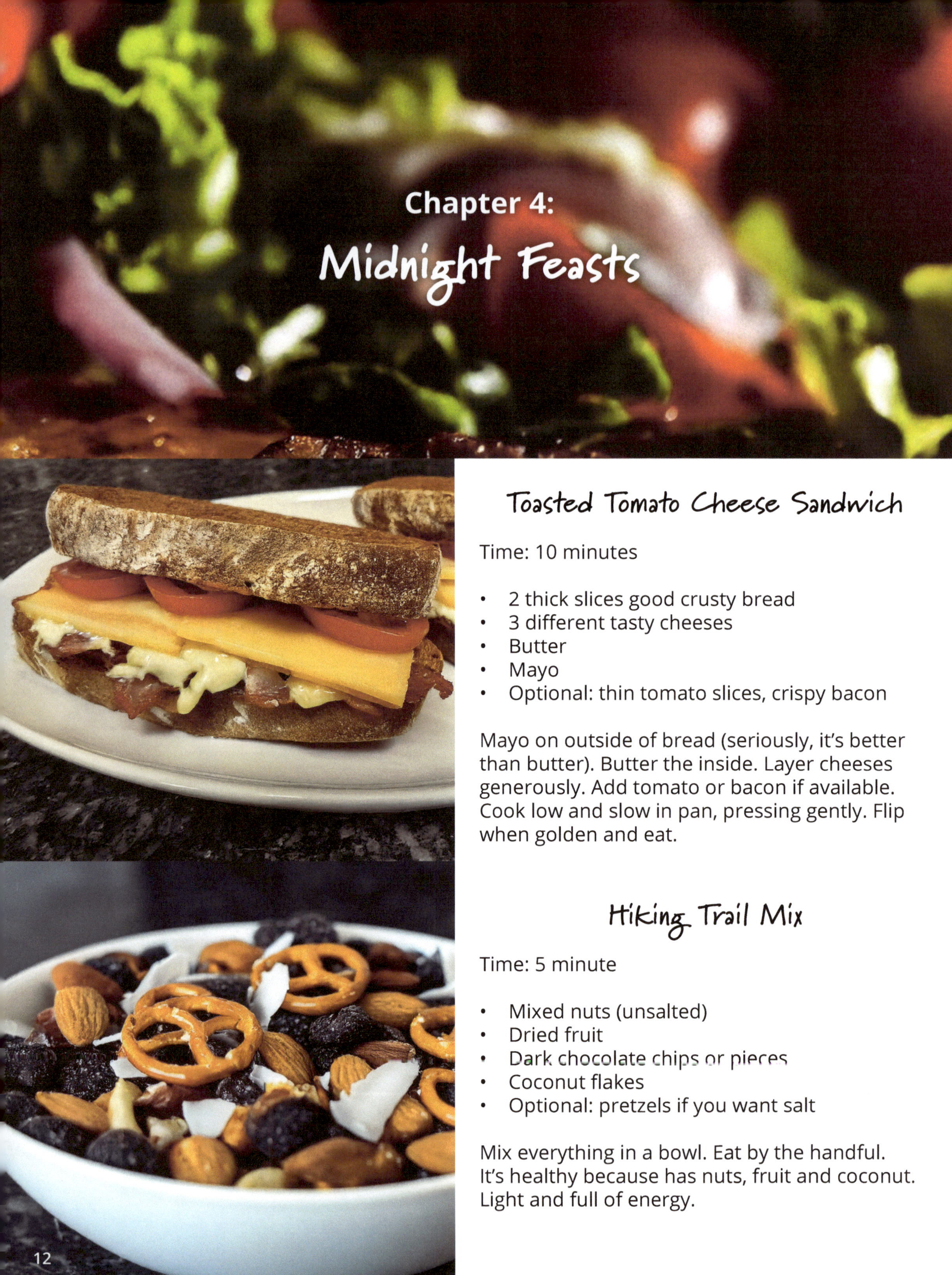

Toasted Tomato Cheese Sandwich

Time: 10 minutes

- 2 thick slices good crusty bread
- 3 different tasty cheeses
- Butter
- Mayo
- Optional: thin tomato slices, crispy bacon

Mayo on outside of bread (seriously, it's better than butter). Butter the inside. Layer cheeses generously. Add tomato or bacon if available. Cook low and slow in pan, pressing gently. Flip when golden and eat.

Hiking Trail Mix

Time: 5 minute

- Mixed nuts (unsalted)
- Dried fruit
- Dark chocolate chips or pieces
- Coconut flakes
- Optional: pretzels if you want salt

Mix everything in a bowl. Eat by the handful. It's healthy because has nuts, fruit and coconut. Light and full of energy.

Loaded Baked Potato

Time: 10 minutes

- Large potato
- Butter
- Sour cream
- Cheese
- Bacon bits
- Chives and broccoli

Microwave potato for 5-6 minutes. Cut open. Load with cheese first and then chopped toppings. Eat hot with a fork while the cheese melts.

Avocado Toast Upgrade

Time: 10 minutes

- Good bread, toasted
- 1 ripe avocado
- Lemon juice
- Tomato and feta cheese sliced
- 1 Egg
- Kick Ass Seasoning or salt and pepper

Mash avocado with salt, pepper, and lemon mixed in. Spread on toast. Add tomato, feta cheese and cooked egg, fried, scrambled on top. Art on toast.

Peanut Banana Crunch

Time: 8 minutes

- 2 slices bread (toasted)
- Peanut butter
- 1 banana, sliced
- Honey
- Optional: granola or crushed cereal for crunch

Spread peanut butter on toasted bread. Add banana slices. Drizzle honey. Add crunch if you want texture. Great in the middle of the night.

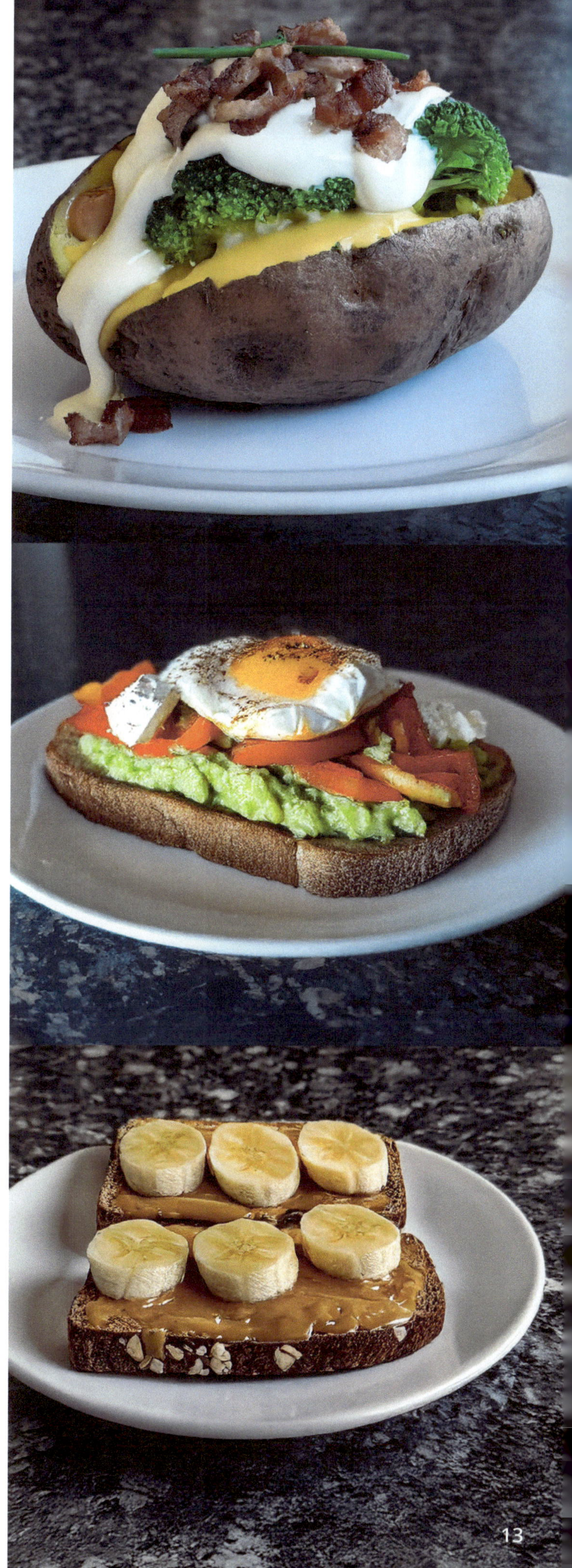

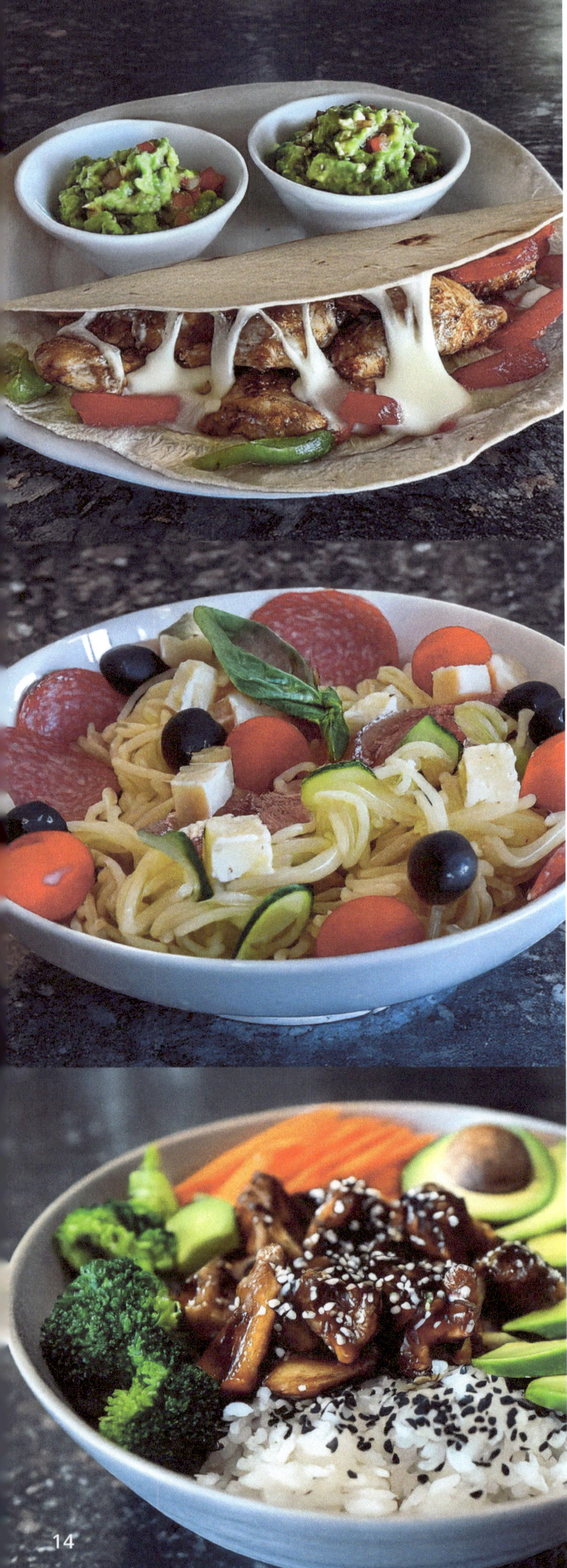

Quesadilla That Rocks

Time: 15 minutes

- 1 Plain tortilla
- Cheese (tasty matured stuff)
- Leftover chicken, beef or lamb
- Salsa or Kick Ass seasoning
- Sour cream
- Peppers sliced
- Guacamole

Put all ingredients in tortilla. Cook in pan until golden and cheese melts. Dip in guacamole and enjoy.

Pasta Salad (Cold)

Time: 15 minutes

- Pasta (any shape)
- Cherry tomatoes
- Cucumber
- Cheese cubes
- Salami,
- Olives
- Italian dressing (Edition 2)

Cook pasta. Rinse with cold water. Mix with everything else. Eat cold. Keeps for days in the fridge.

Rice Bowl Assembly

Time: 15 minutes

- Cooked rice (microwave packets work fine)
- Rotisserie chicken or canned beans
- Frozen vegetables (microwave them)
- Soy sauce
- Avocado,
- Everything seasoning

Cook rice. Heat and add protein and veggies in groups. Drizzle sauce over chicken or beans. Mix as you eat.

Egg Fried Rice (Lazy Version)

Time: 15 minutes

- Microwave rice packet
- 2 eggs, scrambled
- Frozen mixed vegetables
- Soy sauce
- Sesame oil (if you have it)
- Leftover meat, Everything seasoning

Cook rice. Scramble eggs in pan. Add rice, frozen veggies and left over seasoned meat. Add soy sauce and serve when hot.

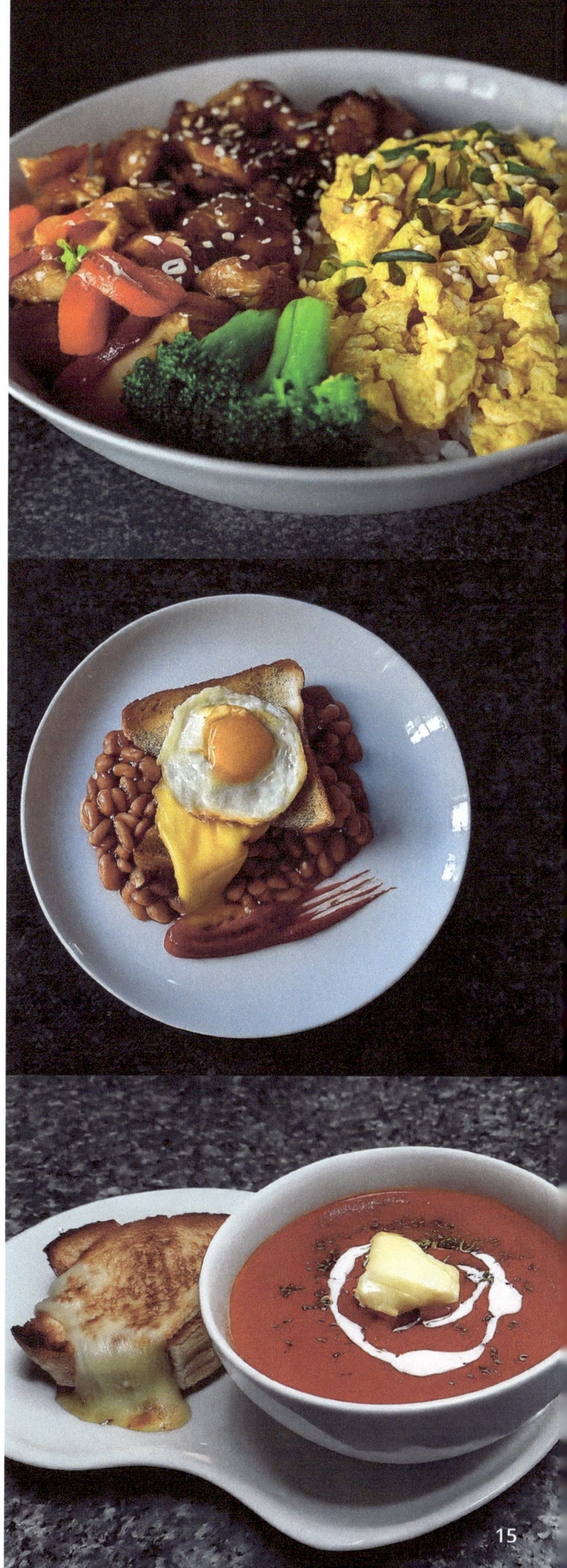

Beans and Toast (Elevated)

Time: 12 minutes

- Fried egg
- Canned beans
- Toast
- Tasty cheese slice
- Hot sauce

Heat beans and pour. Add sliced toast and cheese with a dash of hot sauce for dipping. Top with fried egg for the perfect emergency meal at any hour.

Grilled Cheese and Tomato Soup

Time: 15 minutes

- Canned tomato soup
- 2 slices bread
- Cheese slices
- Sour Cream
- Butter
- Basil or Italian Blend seasoning

Heat soup and add sour cream with seasoning. Make grilled cheese (butter bread, add cheese, cook until golden). Dip sandwich in soup and eat while hot.

Chapter 5

Lazy Spice Blends

Add variety to many of the recipes in this book and other editions using three blends of seasoning.

Everything Seasoning

Mix together:

- 2 tbsp sesame seeds
- 1 tbsp poppy seeds
- 1 tbsp dried garlic flakes
- 1 tbsp dried onion flakes
- 2 tsp coarse salt

Combine and sprinkle on literally everything roasted, fried or BBQ. Good to always have around.

Kick Ass Seasoning

Mix together:

- 1 tbsp chili powder
- 1 tsp cumin
- 1 tsp paprika
- 1/2 tsp garlic powder
- 1/2 tsp onion powder
- 1/4 tsp ground black pepper

Combine and sprinkle on roasted meat, roasted vegetables, eggs, seafood and BBQ stuff.

Italian Blend Seasoning

Mix together:

- 2 tbsp dried basil
- 1 tbsp dried oregano
- 1 tbsp dried parsley
- 1 tsp garlic powder
- 1/2 tsp ground black pepper

Combine and sprinkle on pasta, bread, chicken, beef, lamb and seafood. Usually good on anything considered Mediterranean cuisine.

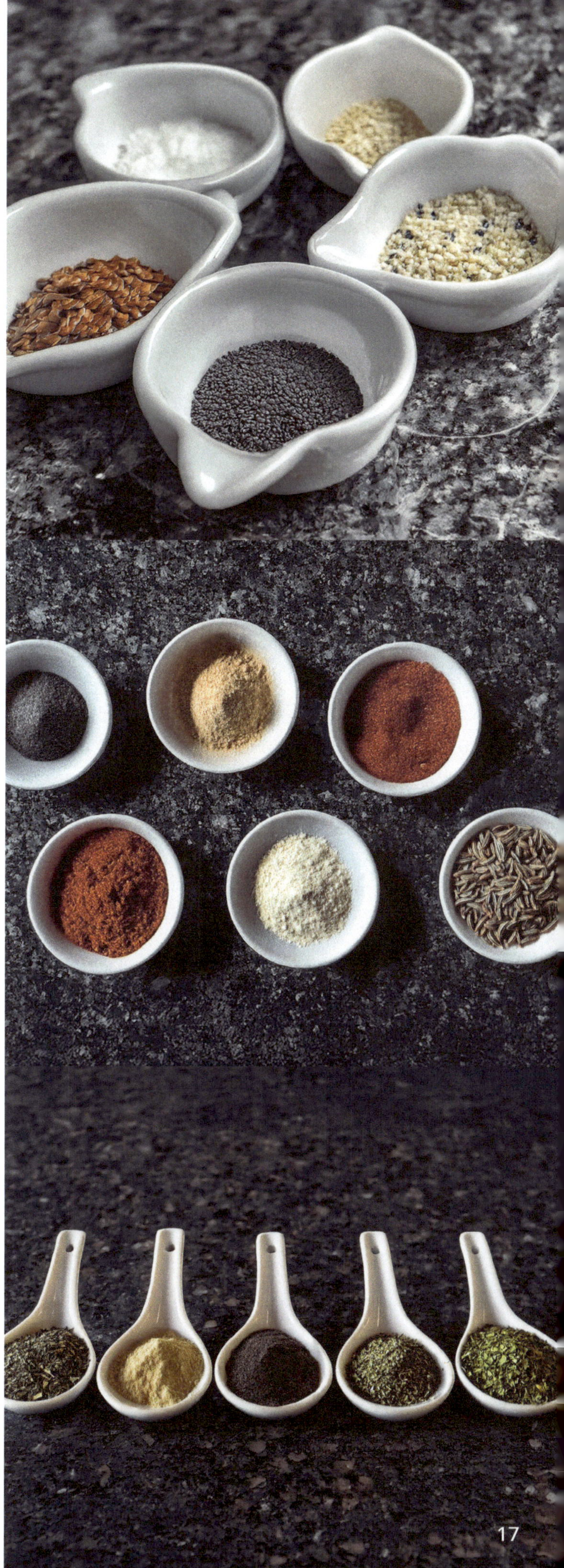

Chapter 6

Zombie Food (it was a big week)

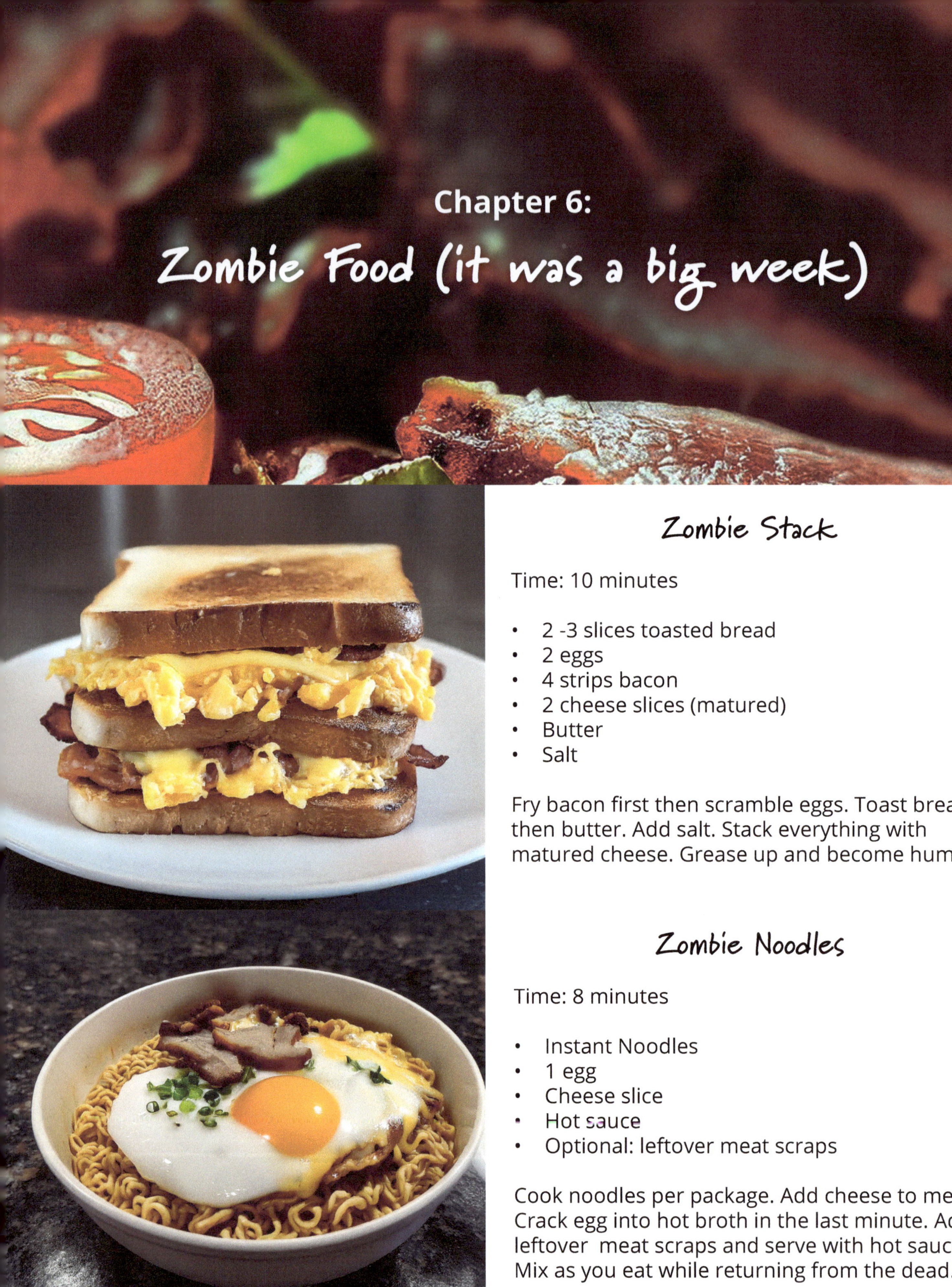

Zombie Stack

Time: 10 minutes

- 2 -3 slices toasted bread
- 2 eggs
- 4 strips bacon
- 2 cheese slices (matured)
- Butter
- Salt

Fry bacon first then scramble eggs. Toast bread, then butter. Add salt. Stack everything with matured cheese. Grease up and become human.

Zombie Noodles

Time: 8 minutes

- Instant Noodles
- 1 egg
- Cheese slice
- Hot sauce
- Optional: leftover meat scraps

Cook noodles per package. Add cheese to melt. Crack egg into hot broth in the last minute. Add leftover meat scraps and serve with hot sauce. Mix as you eat while returning from the dead.

Pita Pocket Rocket

Time: 15 minutes

* Pita bread
* Grilled chicken strips
* Hummus
* Tomato and cucumber diced
* Red onion, sliced thin
* Feta cheese
* Olives

Warm pita. Spread hummus inside. Stuff with vegetables, chicken, feta and olives.

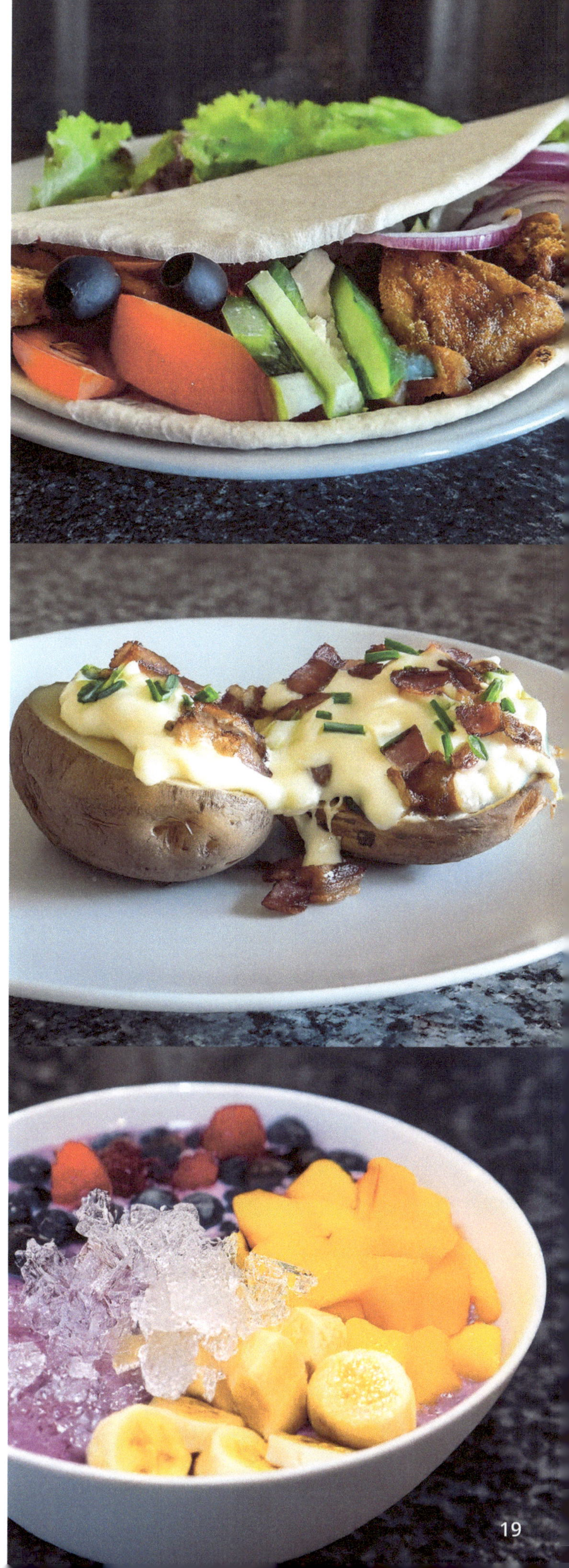

Zombie Potato

Time: 10 minutes

* 1 large potato
* Butter
* Sour cream
* Shredded cheese
* Salt And Cracked Black Pepper
* Bacon bits, chives

Microwave potato for 6-7 minutes. Cut open. Load with butter, sour cream, cheese. Microwave 30 seconds more. Add salt. Shovel into mouth.

Zombie Smoothie

Time: 5 minutes

* Fruit assorted
* Organic berries (fresh or frozen)
* Banana
* 1/4 cup coconut water or sports drink
* Protein powder (if you have it)
* Ice

Blend fruit, berries and coconut water. Top with whole fruit pieces and ice. Consume slowly. The vitamins counteract whatever you did last night.

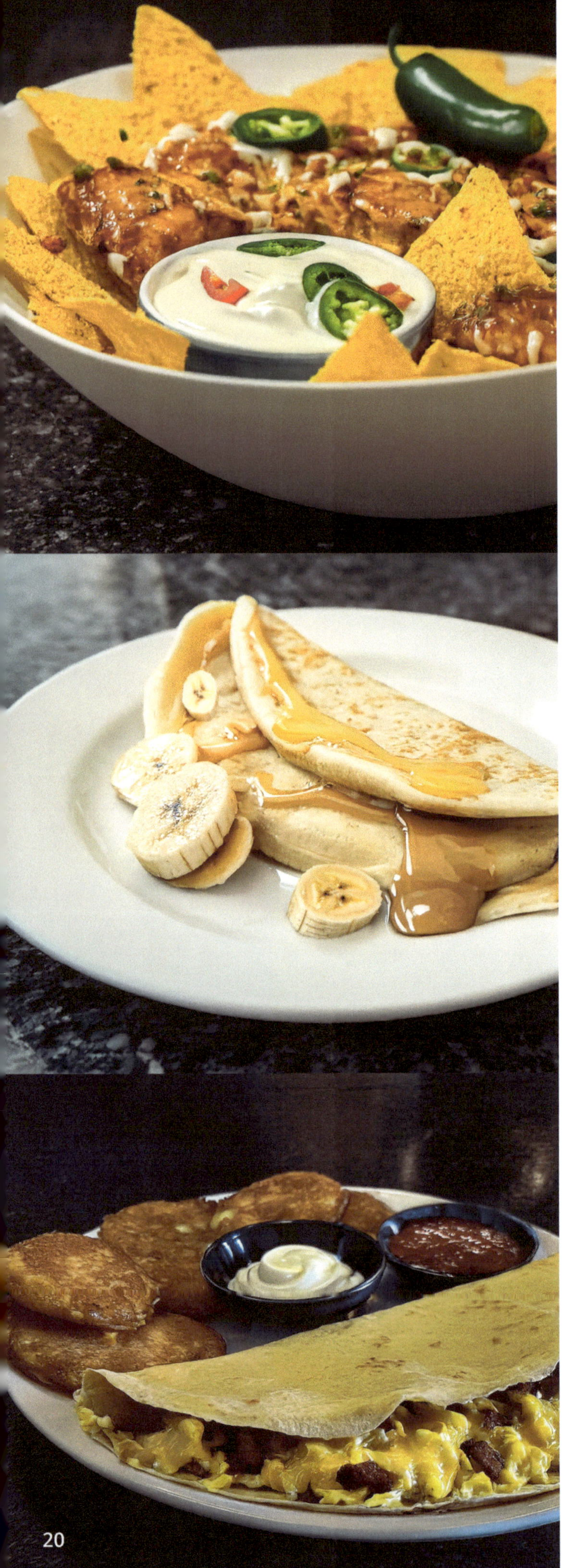

Loaded Zombie Nachos

Time: 12 minutes

- Cheesy Corn chips
- Shredded cheese
- Salsa
- Sour cream
- Jalapenos
- Optional: leftover meat, hot sauce

Pile chips on plate. Cover with cheese. Microwave until melted. Top with everything else. Eat with hands like the night kitchen zombie you are.

Zombie Brain Wrap

Time: 8 minutes

- Flour tortilla
- Peanut butter
- Honey
- Banana slices (optional)
- Butter for pan

Spread peanut butter and honey on half tortilla. Add sliced banana if available. Fold over. Cook in buttered pan until lightly crispy. Drizzle a little honey over.

Zombie Wrap

Time: 15 minutes

- Flour tortilla
- 2 eggs, scrambled
- Shredded cheese
- Hash browns (frozen, microwaved)
- Salsa and sour cream
- Optional: bacon or sausage

Scramble eggs. Heat hash browns. Pile eggs, cheese and meat in the tortilla. Roll up. Serve with hash browns and dips.

Noodle Attack

Time: 15 minutes

- 2 Packs of instant noodles
- 1 egg
- Parmesan cheese
- 1/2 tsp Kick Ass seasoning
- Bacon bits or leftover BBQ meat
- Butter

Separate egg. Cook noodles. Stir in egg white and seasoning, add butter while hot. Top with egg yolk, cheese and pepper. It'll cook slowly from the noodle heat.

Salad Toast For Zombies

Time: 10 minutes

- Crusty thick buttered toast
- Avocado
- Fresh mozzarella
- Tomatoes
- Basil leaves and black pepper
- Balsamic glaze

Spread toast with avocado slices. Add seasoned sliced tomatoes, mozzarella. Drizzle balsamic. Taste the Mediterranean, go back to bed and dream.

Loaded Zombie Sub

Time: 12 minutes

- 1 sub roll
- 4 cheese slices (or shredded cheese)
- Ham
- Tomato slices
- Mayo and garlic flakes (pinch)

Split sub roll lengthwise. Spread mayo on both cut sides. Layer tomato and ham topped with cheese and garlic. Butter outside and cook in pan or grill until golden brown and cheese is melting.

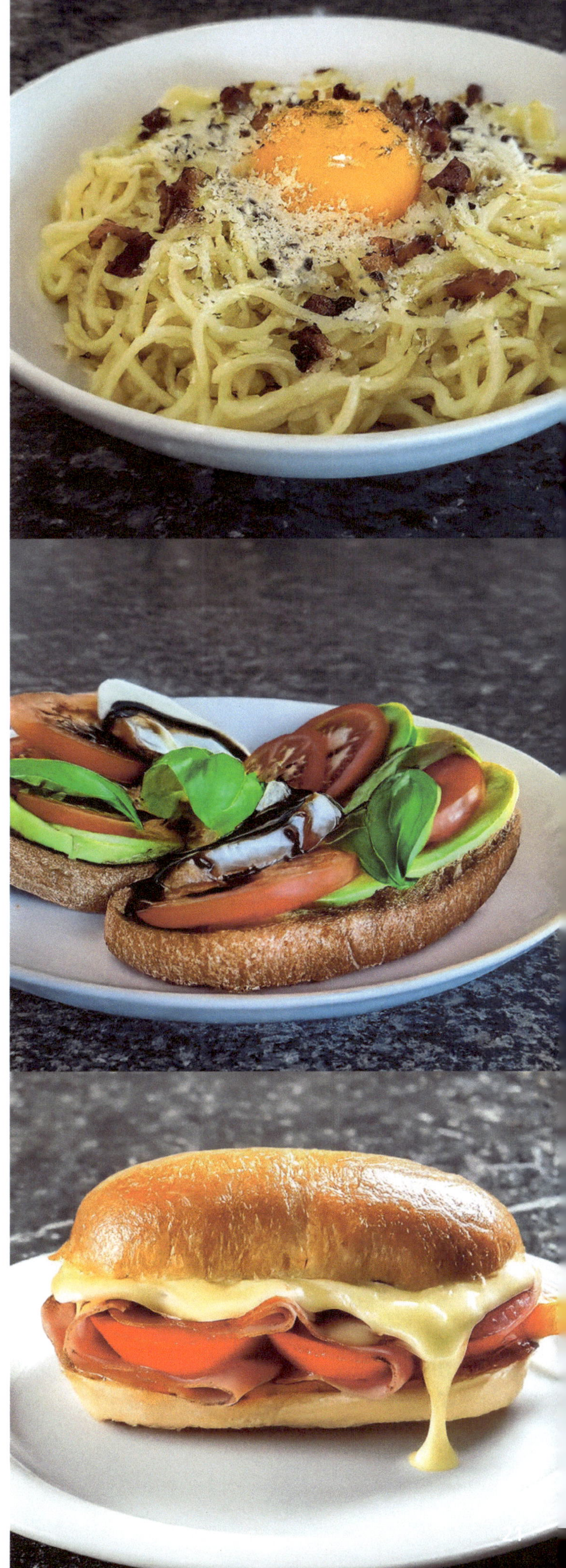

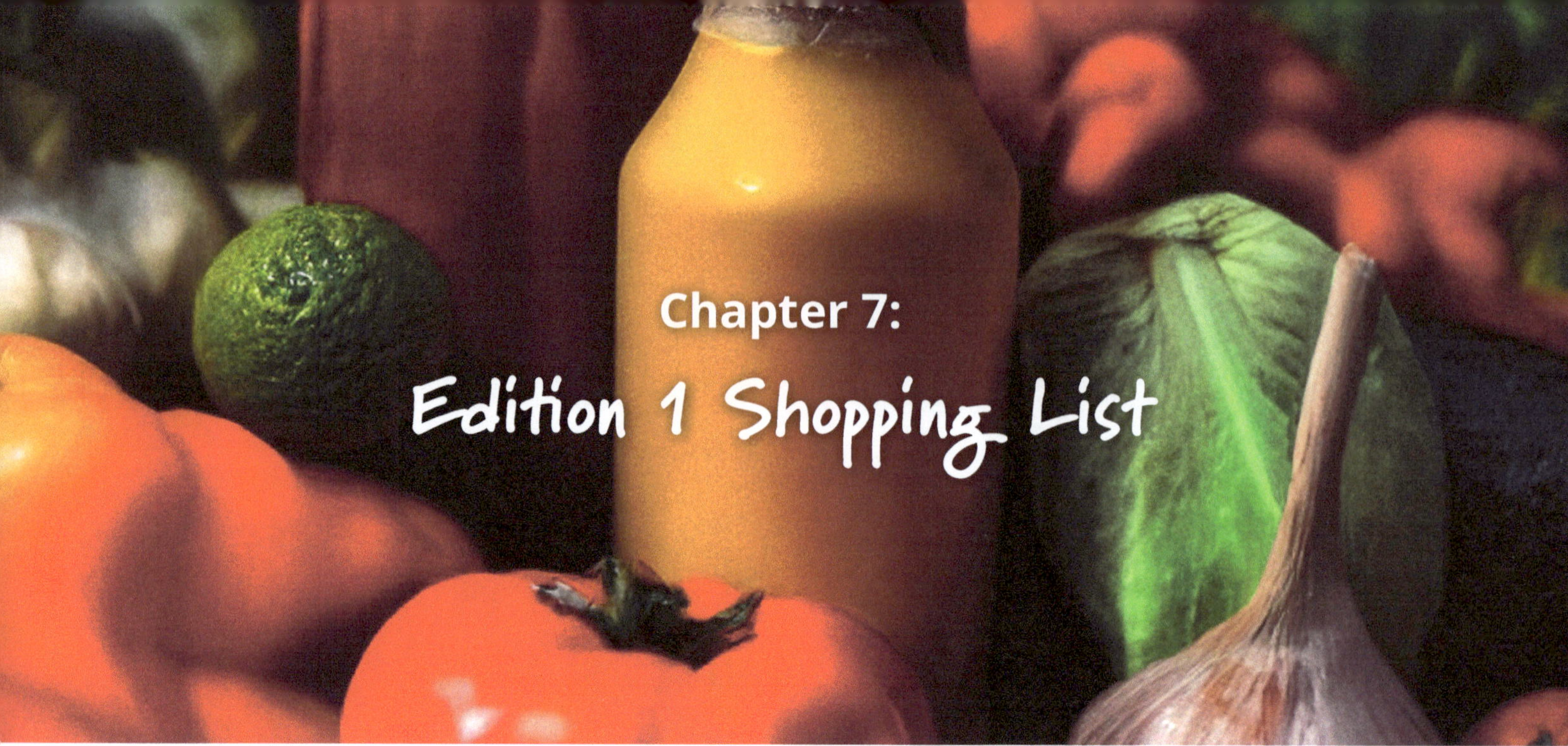

BREADS

- **Sliced bread**
- **Plain or Spinach tortillas**
- Sub rolls
- Bread Rolls
- Croissants
- Pita bread

PROTEINS (The Workhorses)

- **Eggs (must have)**
- **Canned tuna**
- **Canned beans (black, chickpeas)**
- **Rotisserie chicken**
- Deli turkey
- Ham
- Salami
- Pepperoni
- Sliced roast beef
- Pre-cooked bacon
- Frozen meatballs

CHEESE

- **Shredded cheese**
- **Sliced cheddar**
- Swiss cheese
- Mozzarella (sliced and fresh)
- Feta cheese
- Parmesan cheese
- Cream cheese

FRUIT & VEGETABLES (Fresh & Frozen)

- **Lettuce/spinach (bagged is fine)**
- **Tomatoes (cherry and regular)**
- **Cucumber**
- **Bell peppers**
- **Red onion**
- **Bananas**
- **Avocados**
- **Organic berries (fresh or frozen)**
- Shredded carrots
- Coleslaw mix
- Celery
- Lettuce
- Frozen mixed vegetables
- Frozen peas
- Frozen hash browns
- Broccoli
- Fresh basil
- Chives
- Green and red onions
- Frozen fruit for smoothies
- Apples
- Lemons

PANTRY STAPLES

- **Rice (or microwave packets)**
- **Pasta (various shapes)**
- **Instant noodles**
- **Peanut butter**
- **Olive oil**
- **Salt**
- Old-fashioned oats
- Instant couscous
- Canned tomato soup
- Microwave rice packets
- Flour
- Brown sugar
- Vanilla extract
- Chocolate chips
- Honey
- Maple syrup
- Olives
- Pickles

CONDIMENTS & SAUCES

- **Mayo**
- **Butter**
- **Tomato sauce**
- **Olive oil**
- **Soy sauce**
- Mustard hot (yellow)
- Mustard seed
- BBQ sauce
- Marinara sauce
- Tabasco sauce
- Hummus
- Teriyaki sauce
- Sesame oil
- Balsamic glaze
- White wine vinegar
- Horseradish sauce
- Sour cream
- Salsa
- Guacamole
- Coconut water

SPICES & SEASONINGS

- **Garlic powder**
- **Onion powder**
- **Black pepper**
- Chili powder
- Ground cumin
- Paprika
- Red pepper flakes
- Dried basil
- Dried oregano
- Dried parsley
- Italian seasoning
- Sesame seeds
- Poppy seeds
- Dried garlic flakes
- Dried onion flakes
- Coarse salt

BREAKFAST & SNACK ITEMS

- **Your favorite cereals**
- **Greek yogurt**
- **Milk or Tiger Nut Milk**
- Granola
- Mixed nuts
- Chia seeds
- Dried fruit
- Coconut flakes
- Pretzels
- Tortilla chips
- Protein powder (optional)

Shopping Tips:

- Start with the items in **bold** - these appear in multiple recipes
- Rotisserie chicken will save you time
- Pre-cook bacon bits to save time
- Pre-cut vegetables exist to save time
- Buy tortillas in bulk - they freeze well
- Keep eggs, cheese, and bread on hand
- Generic brands work fine for most things
- Keep a hot sauce and 3 x seasoning on hand
- Pickling is a great way to store food
- Frozen bread and wraps can save the day
- Frozen vegetables and fruit are nutritious
- If you're traveling take this book with you

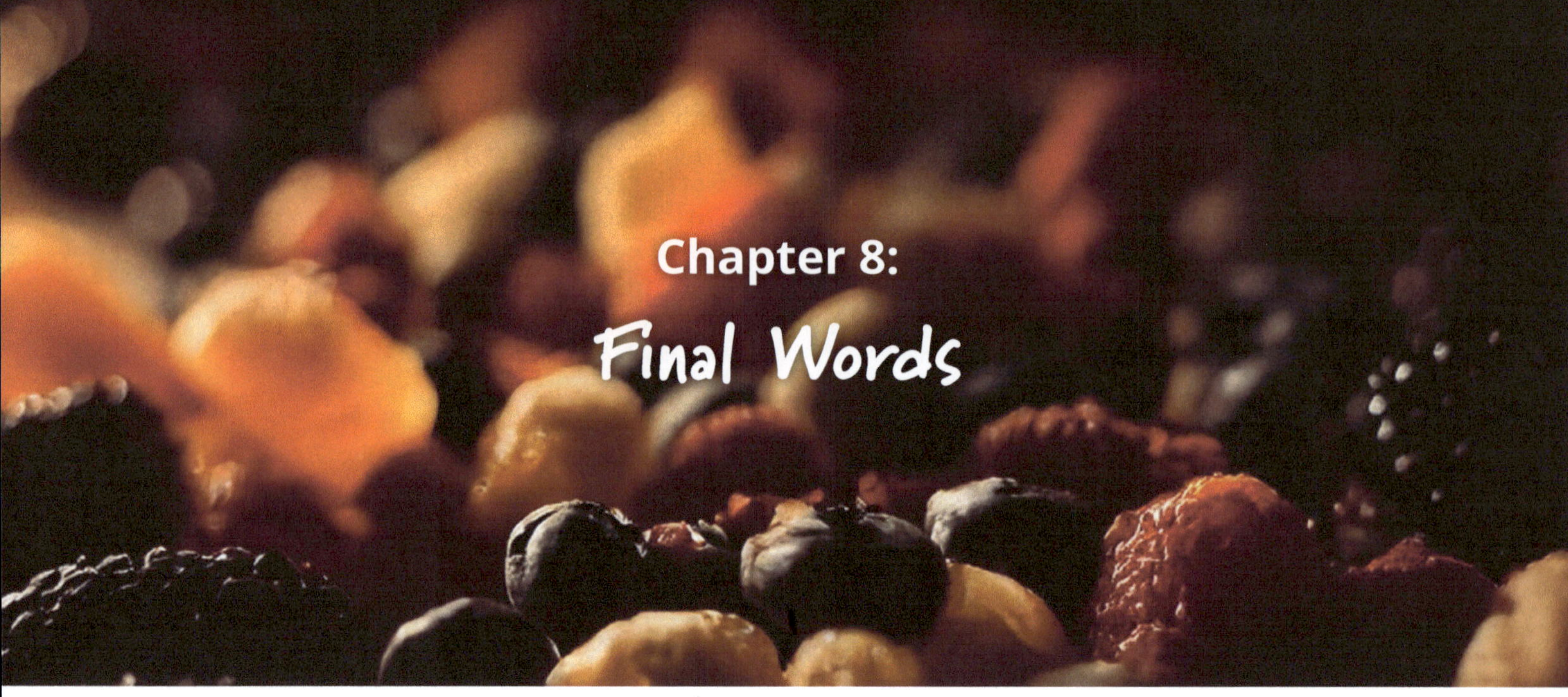

We've all been there, looking in the fridge and thinking, 'I can't be bothered cooking.'

Preparing meals doesn't have to be complicated and with simple combinations using different seasoning and dressings can keep basic meals interesting. Sometimes you just need food that tastes good and doesn't require a PhD in culinary arts. These recipes are for real life when you're busy and exhausted.

Keep your pantry stocked with basics: good bread, tortillas, canned beans, pasta, rice, eggs, cheese, hot sauce, pickles and at least three spices mixes. With these building blocks, you can always make something decent that has variety. And remember: there's no shame in eating cereal for dinner or having a sandwich at 10 AM using BBQ leftovers.

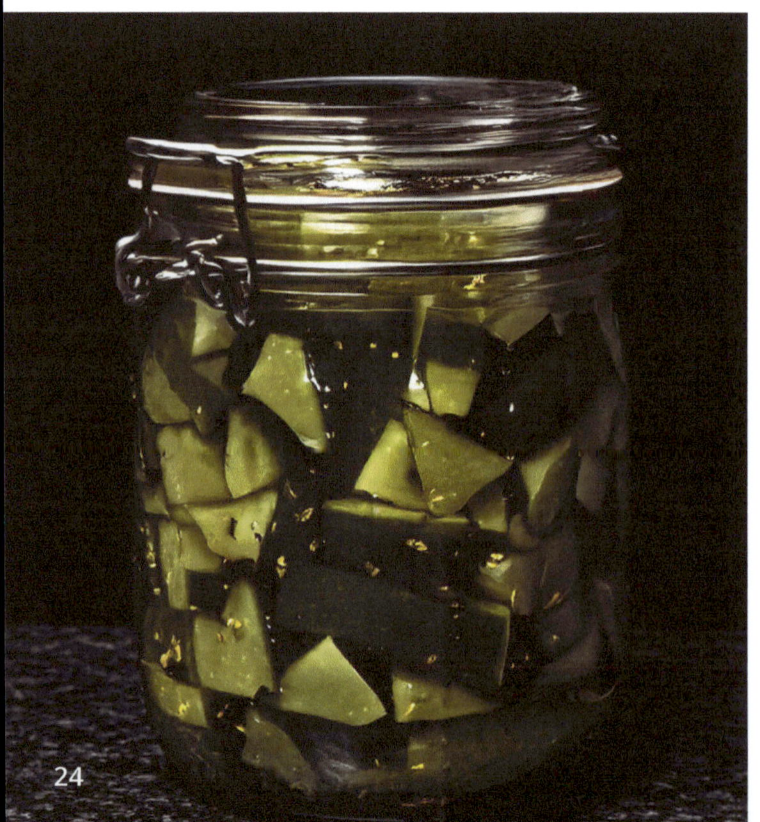

Quick Pickles

Time: Store For Two Days Before Use

- Cucumber thick diced to fill a storage jar
- 3 parts White wine vinegar
- 2 parts Water
- 1 part Sugar
- Salt
- Mustard seed
- Italian Blend seasoning

Add salt to sliced cucumber, rest for thirty minutes. Wash cucumber, add to a jar with sugar, water and white wine vinegar. Add mustard seed and Italian Blend seasoning. Store for two days before use.

Recipe Index

About The Author

Most single professionals would agree that life can be relentless. M. J. Adams has spent many years working in high stake industries that are time dependent so is used to living under the pump and working long hours. Being able to quickly prepare good food with minimal prep and clean up became a necessity which is why this cook book has been published. Good food with minimum prep, cooking and cleanup for hectic lives.

"When I can't be bothered cooking, I still want to eat good food."

M. J. Adams

Edition 2

Recipe Collection For When You Need Good Food
But Can't Be Bothered Cooking.

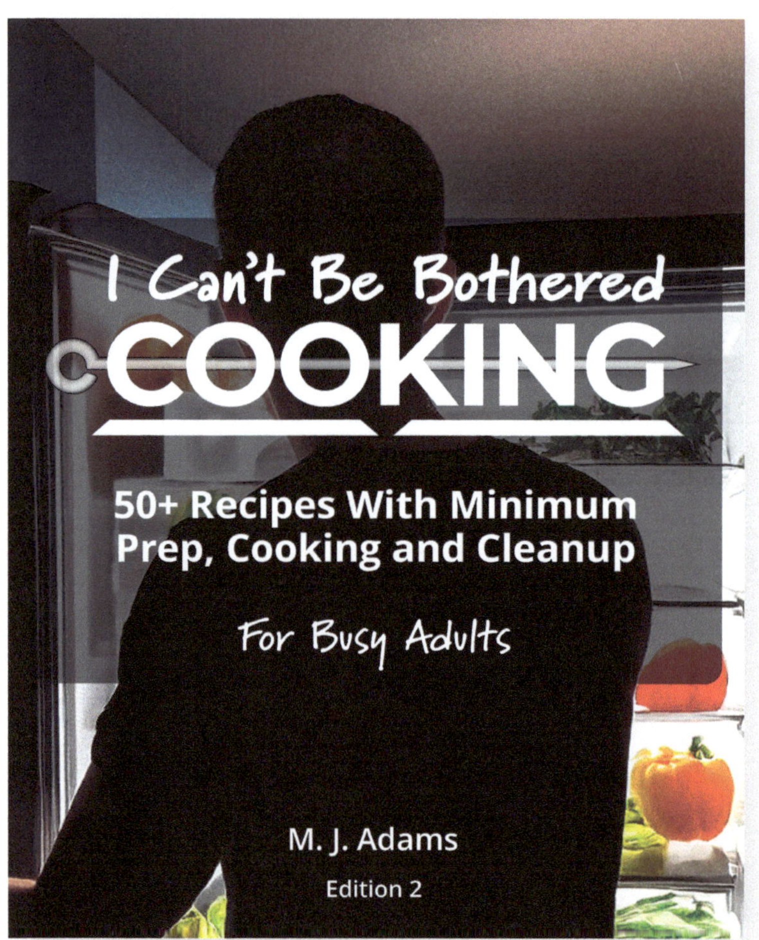

Available From All Good Bookstores

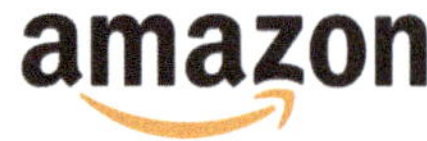

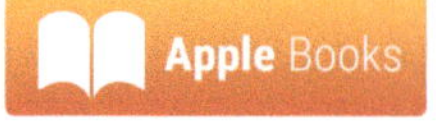